In Dora's Case

Freud—Hysteria—Feminism

Gender and Culture
Carolyn G. Heilbrun and Nancy K. Miller, editors

In Dora's Case

Freud—Hysteria—Feminism

Charles Bernheimer and
Claire Kahane, editors

Columbia University Press
New York 1985

Library of Congress Cataloging in Publication Data

Bernheimer, Charles, 1942–
In Dora's case.

(Gender and culture)
Includes bibliographical references and index.
1. Psychoanalysis—Case studies. 2. Hysteria—Case studies. 3. Feminism—Case studies. 4. Bauer, Ida, 1882–1945. 5. Freud, Sigmund, 1856–1939. 6. Sex (Psychology)—Social aspects—Case studies. 7. Women—Mental health—Case studies. I. Kahane, Claire. II. Title.
RC509.8.B46 1985 616.85'2409 84-19990
ISBN 0-231-05910-8
ISBN 0-231-05911-6 (pbk.)

Columbia University Press
New York

Printed in the United States of America

Clothbound editions of Columbia University Press Books
are Smyth-sewn and printed
on permanent and durable acid-free paper.

GENDER AND CULTURE

A series of Columbia University Press
Edited by Carolyn G. Heilbrun *and* Nancy K. Miller

Breaking the Chain: Women, Theory, and French Realist Fiction,
NAOMI SCHOR

Between Men: English Literature and Male Homosocial Desire,
EVE KOSOFSKY SEDGWICK

In Dora's Case: Freud, Feminism, Hysteria,
CHARLES BERNHEIMER AND CLAIRE KAHANE, EDS.

Contents

Preface

We have standardized all references to the Dora case throughout this book. References, included in the text, are first to the *Standard Edition of the Complete Psychological Works,* translated and edited by James Strachey, 24 vols. (London: Hogarth Press, 1953–1974), abbreviated *SE,* and second to the Collier paperback edition, Philip Rieff, ed. (New York: 1971), abbreviated *C.* Whenever a reference to *The Pelican Freud Library,* vol. 8, *Case Histories I: "Dora" and "Little Hans"* (Harmondsworth: Penguin, 1977) was provided in the original, we have included this additional page number (abbreviated *P*) for the benefit of our British readers. References to Freud's works other than the Dora case are always to the *Standard Edition.* We have generally maintained each author's footnoting style.

Editorial remarks throughout the text are enclosed in brackets.

We had hoped to publish a translation of the dialogue between Catherine Clément and Hélène Cixous that concludes their book *La jeune née* (Paris: 10/18, 1975), to which several of our authors refer, but we could not obtain permission to reprint. A translation by Betsy Wing is scheduled to be published by the University of Minnesota Press in the spring of 1985.

As the length of our bibliography suggests, we had many articles from which to make our selection for this anthology. Certain pieces belonged unquestioningly: Deutsch's because it provides a second psychoanalytic assessment of Dora later in her life; Marcus's because it was the first, and probably is still the best, reading of the case as a literary work; Lacan's because of the reputation of its author and the impact of his reading on subsequent interpreters. Erikson's analysis, although less influential than Lacan's, is also a significant contribution by a major figure in the history of psychoanalysis.

Beyond these four articles, our choice became more difficult. Available studies tend to fall into one of two categories: articles by psychoanalysts, most of which have a clinical orientation, and articles by literary critics, most of which have a feminist orientation. Assuming that our readers would have interests similar to our own, we decided not to reprint articles of a technical nature and to give preference to those analyses that question Freud's assumptions about femininity and female desire. This required leaving out a number of articles that we find suggestive and relevant, in particular those by Alan and Janis Krohn, Jean-Jacques Moscovitz, and Hyman Muslin and Merton Gill. Another piece of considerable interest that we had to omit is historian Hannah Decker's study of Freud's overdetermined choice of the name "Dora." She argues that Freud named his patient not only after his sister's nursemaid, as he explained himself, but also after Dora Breuer, Josef Breuer's youngest daughter. Decker notes similarities in both the lives and the symptoms of Breuer's patient Anna O. and Freud's Dora and in the dynamics of transference and counter-transference in the two cases.

Had we had more space, we would also have liked to include one or more of the articles (by Ann Kaplan, Felicity Oppé, Catherine Protuges, or Jane Weinstock) on the experimental film version of the case, *Sigmund Freud's Dora: A Case of Mistaken Identity*. But since we could not count on many of our readers having seen the film, which was designed to be screened to small groups and followed by a discussion with the filmmakers, we decided to omit these cinematic analyses.

Among the feminist rereadings of the case, which constitute a kind of mini-tradition within the recently constituted field of feminist criticism, a number of authors situate their critiques within the context of contemporary French writing on psychoanalysis and feminism. The articles by Suzanne Gearhart and Jacqueline Rose both address Lacan directly and relate his contribution, more or less critically, to the work of contemporary French feminist theoreticians such as Luce Irigaray, Michèle Montrelay, and Julia Kristeva. Jane Gallop's analysis provides a provocative commentary on the work of Hélène Cixous, her *Portrait de Dora* and her discussions of hysteria with Catherine Clément in *La jeune née*. These three articles thus not only suggest new perspectives on Freud's case but also offer a condensed introduction to some of the most challenging French feminist thinkers.

The remaining five articles display the variety and finesse of the interpretive strategies exercised by contemporary feminist critics. Each offers an original reading of Freud's inscription—through identification, transference, defense, or countertransference—in the drama he is authoring that, both narratively and psychologically, escapes his control.

The editors would like to thank their graduate assistant, Gwen Ashbaugh, for her untiring help in every aspect of putting this anthology together. Joan Cipperman sustained the project by cheerfully giving first priority in her busy schedule to typing the manuscript. Bill Germano and Joan McQuary of Columbia University Press were supportive and enlightened editors. To Nancy Miller and Carolyn Heilbrun we owe special thanks for giving our proposal their support from the start. Elaine Showalter mentioned the idea of a Dora anthology to one of the editors within a few days of the other's proposal of a collaboration on just such a collection. We thank Elaine for her generosity in encouraging us to go ahead with the project. We are grateful to our colleagues David Willbern, Bill Warner and Murray Schwartz for their helpful critical readings of our introduction. Finally, Neil Hertz has assisted us on a number of occasions by offering advice and bibliographical information.

ACKNOWLEDGMENTS

We would like to thank Toril Moi, Jacqueline Rose, and Maria Ramas for permission to reprint their personally copyrighted articles and Dr. Martin Deutsch for the right to reprint his father's article. Other permissions were generously given by the authors and by the following periodicals and presses (see the footnote on the first page of each article for precise references):

Journal of the American Psychoanalytic Association for Erik Erikson's article;
Partisan Review for Steven Marcus's essay;
W. W. Norton and Macmillan/London for the translation by Jacqueline Rose of Lacan's article;
Johns Hopkins University Press for the articles by Gearhart, Collins et al., and Hertz;
Cornell University Press and Macmillan/London for the chapter from Jane Gallop's book, and Cornell University Press for the essay by Madelon Sprengnether.

Introduction
Part One

CHARLES BERNHEIMER

Freud invented psychoanalysis between 1895 and 1900 on the basis of his clinical experience with hysterical patients, nearly all of them women, and of the self-analysis he performed to cure his own hysterical symptoms. Hysteria thus is implicated in psychoanalysis in the sense that the science enfolds the disease within it and is constituted simultaneously with this pathological interiority. Yet psychoanalysis contests this originary implication, insisting on its scientific authority and asserting mastery over hysteria as the illness of the other, typically of the feminine other. Contemporary feminism has put this mastery in question from a variety of perspectives. Certain feminists have declared their solidarity with the protest against familial and social constraints whose repression they see as causing the hysteric's physical ailments (Dora, declares Hélène Cixous, "is the core example of the protesting force of women"),[1] while others have argued that the pronounced bisexuality common to hysterics actually privileges them in terms of Freud's own sexual theory.

Hysteria, psychoanalysis, and feminism thus traverse each other in a complex relation of contestation, implication, and solidarity. This dynamic interplay tends to subvert the distinctions between knowledge and its object, sickness and its cure, sexuality and its repression, history and its fantasy-effects. Thereby an astonishingly productive conflictual field is created to which the contributors to this volume trace an intriguing variety of interpretive maps. To give these maps a historical context, the first part of our introduction offers a brief survey of medical treatments for hysteria and reviews Freud's thinking on the subject up to his writing of the Dora case. The second part investigates some of the reasons for the widespread contemporary interest in this case and provides a critical overview of the approaches adopted in the articles that follow. In a biographical note we give a brief sketch of what is known today about the family of the actual Dora, whose real name was Ida Bauer.

WANDERING WOMBS: A BRIEF HISTORY OF HYSTERIA

For centuries the understanding of hysteria was a prisoner to its etymological origin in the Greek word for uterus. To free it, the great French neurologist Charcot instructed his students to pretend "that the word 'hysteria' means nothing."[2] Charcot hoped thereby not only to encourage his students to find hysterical symptoms in men as well as in women but also to stress the importance of psychic factors in the etiology of the disease. His remark may also be understood as a comment on the extraordinarily elusive character of the disease itself, definitions of which have changed so radically through the ages that to refer to it as a single phenomenon may be no more than a convenient fiction.

Hysteria does indeed have a venerable history. The oldest surviving Egyptian medical papyrus, dating from around 1900 B.C., deals specifically with recommended treatments for hysterical disorders (one illustrative case: " a woman who loves bed; she does not rise and does not shake it"—Veith:3). The cause for such curious behavioral disturbances, as the Egyptians saw it, was the flight of the uterus, which they considered a mobile, independent organism, up and away from its normal position. Cure for this anomalous displacement could be attempted from two directions: the woman's sexual parts could be fumigated with fragrant substances to attract the migratory uterus from below, or vile-tasting and foul-smelling potions could be ingested to drive the deviant womb back from above. These bizarre therapeutic measures, entirely logical within the framework of existing anatomical knowledge, were incorporated into Greek medical literature. Various Hippocratic treatises, moreover, expound the connection, only implied in the Egyptian papyri, between hysteria and "abnormal" sexual activity (including abstinence). They link the upward displacement of the uterus, which was thought to impede the flow of breath, causing convulsions, to a mature woman's deprivation of sexual relations. This is Plato's description in the *Timaeus* (91c):

> The womb is an animal which longs to generate children. When it remains barren too long after puberty, it is distressed and sorely disturbed, and straying about in the body and cutting off the passages of the breath, it impedes respiration and brings the sufferer into the extremest anguish and provokes all manner of diseases besides. (Veith: 7–8)

The recommended treatment here, as well as in the Hippocratic texts, is, quite simply, marriage and pregnancy. Thus was established a diagnosis of female sexual disturbance, and a cure by submission to the yoke of patriarchy (the reproduction of mothering), both of which remained basic to the medical concept of hysteria for centuries to come.

In medieval times, female deviance was interpreted less in the physical terms of uterine disorder than in the supernatural terms of witchcraft and heresy. Although Augustine nowhere writes of hysteria specifically, his belief in witchcraft and demonic possession encouraged his followers to judge the hysteric as someone either willfully evil, and probably in league with the devil, or victimized by witchcraft. A reading of *Malleus Maleficarum* (*Witches' Hammer,* 1494), an immensely popular treatise written by Dominican monks, suggests that the witch mania was largely sustained by virulent misogyny. "What else is woman," exclaim the authors, "but a foe to friendship, an inescapable punishment, a necessary evil, a natural temptation, a desirable calamity, a domestic danger, a delectable detriment, an evil of nature, painted with fair colours!"[3] Thus they consider it entirely natural for women to form alliances with the devil, and the clear implication of the treatise is that all women, being constitutionally inferior, deceitful, and vicious, are witches *in potentia.* Certainly those with hysterical symptoms, such as partial anesthesia, mutism, or convulsions, were to be viewed as under the devil's influence, the question as to whether they were wielders of that influence or its victims being a matter for the courts of inquisition to decide. Catherine Clément persuasively argues that these trials, theatricalized rituals where a mostly male audience enjoyed the spectacle of a woman's demonic possession, evidence of her aberrant otherness, were the precursors of Charcot's famous clinical séances at the Salpêtrière.[4]

In the seventeenth century, Thomas Willis and Thomas Sydenham both questioned the uterine explanation of hysteria and suggested a possible mental origin for the disease. In *Madness and Civilization* Michel Foucault explains why this insight did not open the way for a psychological analysis of hysteria: these doctors conceived the brain in entirely mechanical terms as the distributor or relay station for certain vaguely defined "animal spirits" which, if out of balance, could rapidly traverse corporeal space and attack whatever bodily organ was weakest at the moment (through a mechanism Freud would later call "somatic compliance").[5] Thus, the more solidly dense and firmly organized the internal space of a body, the less vulnerable it will be to hysterical attacks—which explains women's greater susceptibility. "That is why this desease attacks women more than men," writes Sydenham, "because they have a more delicate, less firm constitution, because they lead a softer life, and because they are accustomed to the luxuries and commodities of life and not to suffering."[6]

As Foucault points out, this conception of internal density is clearly invested with moral and ethical connotations. In the eighteenth century these became more pronounced as the notion of "animal spirits" gave way to that of "sympathies" transmitted through the nervous system. Now the delicacy of woman's highly impressionable sensibility, due to the tenuous nature of her nervous disposition, was adduced to explain the hysterical irritation from which she frequently suffered. Implicit in this essentially psychological explanation was the judgment that an excess of sympathetic feeling overcharges the moral capacity of the soul and that the hysteric's suffering may therefore be deserved punishment for her guilty self-indulgence.

It thus becomes apparent that the psychological understanding of hysteria was born in complicity with a moral condemnation of its victims. This complicity is evident even in the work of Philippe Pinel, who is famous for having removed the chains binding insane inmates at the Bicêtre Hospital in Paris and for having insisted on humane treatment for mental patients. In the early nineteenth century, Pinel demonstrated clinically that the behavioral disorders associated with hysteria could not be traced to any organic changes in the brain or nervous system. Their cause was, in his word, "moral," and his method of treatment resembled modern psychotherapy, with the doctor helping the patient, through regular conversations, to probe the origin of her disturbance. However, Foucault's analysis makes clear that Pinel's therapeutic goal was to enforce the homogeneous rule of bourgeois morality, and the asylum as he created it became a juridical space dedicated to the repression of difference and the creation of socially acceptable remorse.[7] In the case of hysterics, whose symptoms Pinel associated with "deviant" sexual conduct (masturbation, prurient stimulation by pornography, irregular menstruation), cure involved, as it had for Plato, Marriage, the Family, and productive Work.

Pinel's brand of paternalistic and normative therapy was congenial to the repressive spirit of the Victorian age, during which, by all accounts, the number of hysterical women patients increased dramatically and their doctors felt increasingly provoked and outraged by what they perceived as female treachery, malingering, and immorality. Indeed, the medical reaction became so violent that extreme remedies such as ovariectomies and clitoral cauterization were advocated by certain specialists in cases of intractable hysteria.

This worsening relation between the hysteric and her physician reflects the peculiarly Victorian intensification of the contradictory expectations that had characterized patriarchal attitudes toward women for centuries.[8] In an increasingly industrialized society, the Victorian woman was looked up to as representative of the purity, order, and serenity of earlier, less anxious times. Gentle, submissive, naive, and good, she was also expected to be strong in her righteousness, perfectly controlled in her decorous conduct, and skilled in her domestic managerial capacities. Faced with this conflict, numerous Victorian women developed unconscious defensive strategies whereby they disavowed the intense anger and aggressive impulses for which the culture gave them no outlet. Thus were generated the conversion reactions, prevalent throughout the latter part of the nineteenth century, whereby women transformed their repressed hostility and desire into physical symptoms that simultaneously acknowledged and disowned those feelings.

Like hysterical phenomena through the centuries, these symptoms made use of conventional ideas, myths, and identities of the dominant culture to gain acceptance for the particular attempt at resolution they unconsciously represented. Since a woman was supposed to be fragile, her falling ill and being confined to the sickbed (here we rejoin the exemplary hysteric of ancient Egypt) was therefore acceptable as an affirmative sign of her femininity, although indeed the action could be interpreted as signifying just the opposite, a rejection of femininity as illness and a hatred of the patriarchy that defined it as such. There was thus a good deal of passive aggression involved in Victorian hysteria, and many of these women expressed their suffering not only by manipulating their relatives but also by provoking their physicians. Hence conflict between the hysteric and her doctor, however well meaning he might be, was to a large degree determined by the cultural presuppositions upheld by both—the doctor from a righteous position of power, the patient from a deviant position of powerlessness. She could always accuse him of desiring her illness, while he could always accuse her of using her illness as a weapon against him.

It was in this emotionally charged medical environment that Charcot, already world famous by the 1880s as a clinical neurologist, began to study hysteria at his Parisian hospital for women, the Salpêtrière, and, as Freud declared, "restored its dignity to the topic [of hysteria]" (*SE* 3:19).[9] Although Charcot maintained that the onset of hysteria followed a psychical trauma, he was less interested in therapeutic methods then in scientific analysis of the disease. He brought to his study a passion for careful observation and orderly classification, which also became Freud's modes of gathering knowledge. Freud described Charcot as a seer, a "*visuel,*" not a reflective man but one who observed doggedly until an order emerged from his disparate impressions and he was able to define a nosological type "characterized by the constant combination of certain groups of symptoms" (*SE* 3:12). Using this pragmatic method, he found four stages in every hysterical attack, three categories of hysterical stigmata, and twenty hysterogenic zones on the twenty-year-old female body.

But it was Charcot's controversial method of using hypnotism to produce and remove hysterical symptoms that had the greatest immediate impact on Freud. Charcot became convinced that susceptibility to hypnotism indicated that the subject was potentially hysterical. Hence he considered the hypnotic trance and the hysterical crisis to be essentially equivalent phenomena. This misguided belief was furthered by overzealous assistants who, it is now thought, probably conditioned his patients by implanted suggestion to respond according to their chief's expectations. The demonstrations at the famous *leçons du mardi* were immensely successful spectacles, at least for the professional men who, like Freud, crowded into Charcot's clinic to gaze, with some of the master's own scoptophilia, at the coached performances of his specimen hysterics. The sexual politics of the situation are dramatically revealed in a well-known lithograph, of which a copy hung in Freud's consulting room, that shows an attractive young female patient leaning back into the arms of Charcot's disciple Babinski, the top of her dress down around her waist, her bodice exposed and shoulders bare, while Charcot, standing stolidly next to her, lectures to his attentive male audience. However this staging may have influenced Freud's views of the role of science in the arena of sexual difference, it is clear that Charcot's hypnotic theater strikingly demonstrated to him the existence of radical dissociative trends splitting the consciousness of hysterics, often in terms of socially commendable and socially censurable roles. Through that split Freud gained an initial glimpse onto the "other scene" on which he would eventually stage his discovery of the unconscious.

FREUD'S EVOLUTION FROM CATHARSIS TO PSYCHOANALYSIS

After returning from Paris in 1886 and setting up his own practice in Vienna, Freud continued to publish papers in the field of his professional training, neurology. Meanwhile he was struggling to distinguish physiological from psychological factors in the pathologies of the neurotics who constituted the majority of his patients. Dismissing currently recommended methods of treatment, such as hydrotherapy and electrotherapy, as ineffective, he began using hypnosis, first with therapeutic suggestion, then increasingly as a means to provoke recollection of the emotional conflicts that had originally given rise to the symptoms. He was encouraged to move in this direction by the experience of an older colleague, Josef Breuer, who had told Freud even before the latter's trip to Paris about a case of hysteria he had treated between 1880 and 1882, the famous case of Anna O. (the pseudonym for Bertha Pappenheim, who became the first German social worker and an active feminist). Under deep hypnosis, this patient, who had "presented a variegated picture of paralyses with contractures, inhibitions, and states of mental confusion" (*SE* 20:20), of her own accord began to describe the details surrounding the first appearance of particular symptoms, all of which, as Freud commented in his *Autobiographical Study* of 1925, "went back to moving events which she had experienced while nursing her father; that is to say, her symptoms had a meaning and were residues or reminiscences of those emotional situations" (*SE* 20:20).

Without the benefit of the stage-directing Charcot's patients received, Anna O. made a spectacle of herself as a means of dramatizing through her body, of converting from the psychic to the physical, the tension she felt between her guilt and ambivalence about her father's death and her desire to escape the strangulating demands of a repressive, patriarchal, bourgeois family. Then, in the context of her therapy with Breuer, she discovered the method of her own treatment, which she called "the talking cure" and Breuer "the cathartic method": she translated her conversion symptoms into the narrative of their origin, thereby undoing them. This translation, as Dianne Hunter has recently stressed,[10] involved the movement not only from body language to verbal expression but also from multilingualism to a single language. For among her symptoms had been an inability to understand or communicate in her native German and a tendency to speak in one or more foreign tongues, in sequence or, at times of extreme anxiety, in an unintelligible mixture. This disruptive polylingualism, Hunter argues, may reflect a refusal of the cultural identity inscribed in the order of (coherent) German discourse and an unconscious desire, become conscious in certain contemporary feminist writers, to explode linguistic conventions. Particularly in regard to the dynamics of Freud's later involvement with Dora, it is significant to note that Anna O.'s successful elaboration of a coherent narrative of her past coincided with the creation of an intensely eroticized transference and countertransference between doctor and patient: Anna O. staged an hysterical childbirth and Breuer consequently broke off the treatment and repressed the factor of mutual attraction in his account of the case.

Partly because he experienced difficulty in hypnotizing his patients, partly because he felt that conscious recollection in a state of "concentration" (aided by the physician's manual application of pressure to the patient's forehead) would produce longer-lasting results, Freud gradually gave up using hypnosis in his therapy. Most crucial in this decision, however, was his increasing conviction, born of his attentive listening (Freud privileged the aural as much as Charcot the visual), that apparently wandering thoughts produced by his patients when encouraged to remember the circumstances of their symptoms' origin were actually guided and determined by some definite psychic agency. His patients' avoidances and meanderings, their "free" associations, thus forced him to confront a phenomenon crucial to his discovery of repression and previously obscured by his use of hypnosis—namely, the patient's resistance to unpleasurable ideas and his or her defense against their articulation. As so often in his career, Freud was able in this instance to take what first appeared as an obstacle to treatment and transform it into a means of achieving progress. The interpretation of resistance became his essential analytic tool in the gradual unveiling of unconscious motivation. He also began to appreciate the function of transference in the treatment, although at this time he did not consider it an essential part of the therapeutic relationship but rather a localized "false connection" or displacement of affect to be treated "in the same way as the old symptoms" (*SE* 2:303), that is, by revealing that the physician had been made the object of a long-repressed wish.

The volume Freud published with Breuer in 1895, *Studies on Hysteria,* reflects the transitional state of Freud's thinking at this point. It consists of a theoretical introduction, "On the Psychical Mechanism of Hysterical Phenomena," written jointly by Breuer and Freud and first published separately in 1893, Breuer's case history of Anna O., four case histories by Freud, a theoretical section by Breuer in which he propounds his idea that hysteria originates in certain unusual "hypnoid" mental states (Freud later disclaimed this notion entirely), and a long final chapter by Freud entitled, "The Psychotherapy of Hysteria." Although many crucial psychoanalytic terms are used in this work ("the unconscious," "repression," "defense," "conversion," "transference"), Freud remained uneasy about abandoning the search for a physiological explanation of psychopathological states. Indeed, his postulation of a "principle of constancy" whereby affect is discharged so as to maintain a constant quantity of excitation within the psychic apparatus derives from an essentially physiological and materialist theory of dynamic pressures. And immediately after the publication of the *Studies* Freud wrote what now appears a desperate, albeit brilliant, last-ditch effort to resolve the mind-body duality on the basis of neurophysiology, the long unpublished "Project for a Scientific Psychology."

What one might call, using his own term, Freud's "resistance" to psychology was linked to his mistrust of the novelistic efforts his accounts of case histories required of him. At the outset of his discussion of the case of Fräulein Elisabeth von R., his first full-length analysis of a hysteria (1892–1894), Freud wrote:

> I have not always been a psychotherapist. Like other neuropathologists, I was trained to employ local diagnoses and electro-prognosis, and it still strikes me myself as strange that the case histories I write should read like short stories and that, as one might say, they lack the serious stamp of science. I must console myself with the reflection that the nature of the subject is evidently responsible for this, rather than any preference of my own. The fact is that local diagnosis and electrical reactions lead nowhere in the study of hysteria, whereas a detailed description of mental processes such as we are accustomed to find in the works of imaginative writers enables me, with the use of a few psychological formulas, to obtain at least some kind of insight into the course of that affection. (*SE* 2:160–61)

Thus Freud finds himself implicated inextricably in the complexities of narrative creation. He tells the stories of the stories told him—which is not the same as retelling the original stories—and must articulate at this level of meta-narrative a discourse revealing scientific truth. Moreover, the sheer complication of the processes to be represented at this meta-level forces him to resort to a language of similes ("all of which have only a very limited resemblance to my subject and which, moreover, are incompatible with one another"—*SE* 2:291). So science, in this matter of psychology, often speaks in the figures of poetry. And since such figuration, as Freud noted in 1897, has much in common with hysterical fantasies ("The mechanism of poetry [creative writing] is the same as that of hysterical phantasies"—*SE* 1:256), one might argue that Freud's ambivalence about the literary aspect of his work reflects his uneasy awareness of his own hysterical potential.

There was, however, a fundamentally reassuring aspect to his enterprise: he was convinced that, no matter how metaphorical his language might become, the processes he was attempting to describe were in themselves strictly logical. And they were just as logical, he claimed, in hysterics as in normal people, the hysteric having simply deflected, blocked, or fragmented a logical train of thought, that is, a linear narrative, that the analyst can help her or him reconstruct. "Once we have discovered the concealed motives, which have often remained unconscious," Freud comments, "and have taken them into account, nothing that is puzzling or contrary to rule remains in hysterical connections of thought, any more than in normal ones" (*SE* 2:294). Thus Freud liberated hysterics from the stigma of degeneracy so long attached to them and defined their illness as an extreme mode of something we all do: forgetting the past. "*Hysterics suffer mainly from reminiscences*" (*SE* 2:7), he stressed, their suffering being due to a selective blockage of memory.

It now became crucial to discover whether any one particular object of memory, repressed and reactivated at a later stage, could be the originating cause of hysteria. In their "Preliminary Communication" of 1893, Freud and Breuer admit to having "done no more than touch upon the aetiology of hysteria" (*SE* 2:17), and in their preface to the volume of 1895 they state that reasons of professional confidence have forced them "to produce very incomplete evidence in favour of our view that sexuality seems to play a principal part in the pathogenesis of hysteria as a source of psychical traumas and as a motive for 'defence'—that is, for repressing ideas from consciousness" (*SE* 2:29). Although in his theoretical contribution Breuer actually asserts this thesis in stronger terms than Freud ever uses in the *Studies,* stressing the pathological effects of early sexual repression in girls, Freud's ideas about sexuality developed so rapidly after 1895 that Breuer, once burnt already in the Anna O. case, apparently felt that he could no longer follow his younger friend's lead. Yet, as Freud notes in his *Autobiographical Study,* "in deriving hysteria from sexuality" he was not so much entering new territory as "going back to the very beginnings of medicine and following up a thought of Plato's" (*SE* 20:24). For the Viennese scientist, however, it was not a wandering womb that provoked hysteria but the roving hands of various male seducers.

Freud's papers of 1896 paint a frightening picture of contemporary sexual life in which prepubescent children are regularly the victims of adult sexual molestation. The assailants are most often "nursemaids, governesses, and domestic servants, to whose care children are only too thoughtlessly entrusted" (*SE* 3:164), but they may also be other children, mostly brothers who have been seduced by servants and have had their libido prematurely awakened. More disturbing yet, they can be older family members, fathers, and uncles. Repeatedly denying that any hereditary predisposition could be involved in the frequent occurrence of what one might call "family neuroses," Freud insists that "the logical structure of the neurotic manifestations" (*SE* 3:165) *always* leads back to childhood sexual trauma. The circle of abuse is perfectly vicious: "In one of my cases," Freud writes, "a brother, a sister, and a somewhat older male cousin were all of them ill. From the analysis which I carried out on the brother, I learnt that he was suffering from self-reproaches for being the cause of his sister's illness. He himself had been seduced by his cousin, and the latter, it was well known in the family, had been the victim of his nursemaid" (*SE* 3:165). Freud accounts for the different consequences of seduction for boys and girls in that "the natural sexual passivity of women explains their being more inclined to hysteria" (*SE* 1:228), while men's active role inclines the boy victims of sexual abuse to obsessional neurosis. In the hysteric,

Freud argues, the memory of a passive sexual seduction in early childhood is repressed and remains like a foreign body in the unconscious until reanimated at puberty, when it may either be converted immediately into a symptom or once again repressed as unacceptable to a now sexually aware consciousness. Reactivated in adulthood with the accompanying conflicted sexual feelings, it then finds dramatic expression in a symptom that compromises between the desire to express sexuality and the resistance against it.

This "theory of a foreign body and a splitting of consciousness," Freud observed to Fliess in 1897, is "identical to . . . the medieval theory of possession, held by the ecclesiastical courts (*SE* 1:242). Ordering a *Malleus Maleficarum* for careful study (see *SE* 1:243), Freud at this point is pursuing a "parallel with witchcraft" that casts the seducers in the role of the devil, a casting that, even as it implies moral judgment, simultaneously suggests that the drama might be a delusive psychic creation.

But by 1897 Freud's analyses had convinced him that these devils were, in the majority of cases, "close relatives, a father or a brother" (*SE* 1:246). In order to understand how Freud could have come to this conviction, it is helpful to look beyond his accounts of the particular abuses suffered by his patients to what Steven Marcus has called "the sexual climate of gloom, frustration, fear, and muted despair" that prevailed in bourgeois Vienna at the end of the nineteenth century.[11] As Freud himself portrays the situation in his early letters to Fliess, venereal disease is rampant (and often displays the same symptomatology as hysteria), the prevalant practice of *coitus interruptus* threatens to destroy the marriage relation, masturbation is reducing potency and causing neurasthenia. Bourgeois fathers and brothers regularly seduce the maids in their households, thereby offering as fantasy material to their wives, daughters, and sisters degraded models of female sexuality as servitude or prostitution (see *SE* 1:248).[12] "The maid is the repressed of the mistress," comments Hélène Cixous.[13] Given this decadent, anxiety-ridden sociosexual atmosphere, it is perhaps not so surprising that Freud should have believed that fathers would exploit their own children for sexual gratification.

He had, moreover, the example of one of his own dreams to suggest that even he was not immune to incestuous wishes. He reported the dream to Fliess in a letter of May 1897:

Not long ago I dreamt that I was feeling over-affectionately towards Mathilde [Freud's eldest daughter, aged eleven at this time], but her name was "Hella," and then I saw the word "Hella" in heavy type before me. The solution is that Hella is the name of an American niece whose photograph we have been sent. Mathilde may have been called Hella because she has begun weeping so bitterly recently over the Greek defeats [in the Greco-Turkish war of 1896–1897]. She has a passion for the mythology of ancient Hellas and naturally regards all Hellenes as heroes. The dream of course fulfills my wish to pin down a father as the originator of neurosis and put an end to my persistent doubts. (*SE* 1:206).

Here Freud at once exposes and masks his sexual attraction to his prepubescent daughter. By interpreting his dream as a confirmation of a purely theoretical desire, he displaces his incestuous impulse into the realm of theory, where his particular guilt becomes that of "a father." Theory thus appears as the locus of wish fulfillment, the means through which Freud exonerates himself from a guilty complicity in male fantasies of seduction.

A few months later Freud had come to a theoretical conclusion that served to exculpate him along with the entire group of middle-class fathers: the hypothesis of infantile sexuality. In the famous letter to Fliess of Septmber 21, 1897, in which Freud declares, "I no longer believe in my *neurotica,*" he gives as one of the reasons for rejecting the seduction theory "surprise at the fact that in every case the father, not excluding my own, had to be blamed as a pervert (*SE* 1:259). By determining that seduction scenes are infantile wish fulfillments, fantasies rather than memories, Freud reverses the direction of erotic energy. Seduction now originates with the child's perverse desire, stimulated by autoerotic activity, of which the parent is no more than the passive object. The adult, of course, does not thereby escape guilt—his unconscious harbors memories of his own infantile incestuous wishes—but this guilt is retrospective (in relation to his parents), rather than contemporary (in relation to his children).

Freud's abandonment of the seduction theory has recently come under attack by Jeffrey Masson and certain other revisionists who see this shift from external event to internal invention as a defensive retreat from reality and history.[14] However much Freud may have been tempted by such a retreat, the position he adopted is far more complex than these revisionists allow. William Warner, in a subtle analysis of this issue, argues convincingly that "Freud never accepts the idea that fantasy carries forward so much fictive revision that all contact with an 'actual event' disappears."[15] Memory and fantasy supplement and subvert each other in such an equivocal and undecidable fashion that no single origin, be it an empirical event or an unconscious desire, can ever be conclusively determined. Thus Freud, in his paper on screen memories (1899), tells of his having had to defend the genuineness of a childhood memory his patient wanted to interpret as a suppressed fantasy. "This cannot occur," Freud objects, "unless there is a memory-trace the content of which offers the phantasy a point of contact—comes, at it were, half way to meet it" (*SE* 3:318). This halfway point where the trace of what is outside the psyche meets the projections of what is inside corresponds, Warner suggests, to the middle space of language, the medium of psychoanalysis.

Having realized that "there are no indications of reality in the unconscious, so that one cannot distinguish between the truth and fiction that is cathected with affect (*SE* 1:260), Freud was on the verge of discovering the Oedipus complex. On October 15, 1897, he announced to Fliess: "I have found, in my own case too, falling in love with the mother and jealousy of the father, and I now regard it as a universal event of early childhood" (*SE* 1:265). The context for this momentous discovery was the self-analysis (so designated by him) that Freud undertook for approximately three years, beginning in the summer of 1897. Most of what we know about this analysis comes from the letters Freud wrote during the period to Wilhelm Fliess, a nose and throat specialist who functioned in this relationship somewhat like a therapist in the transference. Freud treated Fliess as an idealized version of himself, using their correspondence and periodic meetings (which he called congresses) to try out his latest insights, theoretical speculations, and perhaps most importantly, analyses of dreams. Something of a theoretical madman, Fliess diagnosed a "nasal reflex neurosis" with widely distributed symptoms whose etiology he associated, surprisingly enough, with genital disturbances, and he devised an elaborate numerical system to demonstrate that a precise law of periodicity, related to the menstrual period, governed all human and animal conduct. For years Freud took these wild ideas seriously, so happy was he to have an eager and enthusiastic listener and correspondent, and they may well have influenced his later conceptions of the upward displacement of genital stimulation and of the repetition compulsion.

Freud's need to idealize Fliess, meetings with whom he looked forward to "as to a slaking of hunger and thirst,"[16] long blinded him to the transference aspects of his friendship and may have delayed his realization of the critical importance of transference in psychoanalytic treatment. In a letter written a few months before the friends' last meeting, however, Freud hints at the submerged erotic component of their relationship: "There can be no substitute for the close contact with a friend which a particular—almost a feminine—side of me calls for." This remark suggests that Freud's unconscious transference managed to dissolve what he called in a late essay "the rebellious overcompensation of the male [that] produces one of the strongest transference-resistances" (*SE* 23:252), that is, the resistance against adopting a passive attitude toward another man. Thus Freud's refusal to "repudiate femininity," a repudiation that he later called the bedrock of psychoanalysis (*SE* 23:252), appears to have been essential not only to the early stages of his self-analysis but to the entire set of discoveries he made in the decisive years between 1895 and the beginning of the Dora analysis in October 1900.

No sooner had Freud encouraged his patients to free associate than they had spontaneously been moved to recount their dreams, a phenomenon whose importance for an understanding of psychic processes he was quick to appreciate. He began to analyze his own dreams in 1895 (the date of the famous dream of Irma's injection), or perhaps even earlier, and sketched out a first approach to a coherent theory of dreams in the "Project." But it was not until the time of his self-analysis that dreams emerged as the human productions that most clearly proved the continuity between the normal and the pathological.

The key is the similarity between the formation of dreams and of symptoms, both being generated through the mechanisms of condensation and displacement and both functioning as wish fulfillments. "The dream pattern is capable of the most general application" he told Fliess in January 1899, "and the key to hysteria as well really lies in dreams" (*SE* 1:276). Indeed, it is in the analysis of his own dreams that Freud had searched in the foregoing years for a resolution to what in 1897 he called "my own hysteria" (*SE* 1:262), and in the 1908 preface to the second edition of *The Interpretation of Dreams* he says that writing that book (in 1898 and 1899) was "a portion of my own self-analysis, my reaction to my father's death" (*SE* 4:xxvi) (which had occurred in 1896). Freud's symptoms involved a combination of psychosomatic manifestations (migraine, digestive disturbances, a nasal infection on which Fliess operated, chronic fatigue) and psychic disturbances (a mild train phobia, certain inhibitions, sudden changes of mood, obsessive ideas concerning death, above all fits of depression and anxiety). Unfortunately, Freud nowhere gives a diagnosis of these symptoms, most of which passed away before 1900, but they were no doubt related not only to his father's death but also, among other factors, to anxiety about his paucity of patients, uncertainty about his ability to cure those he had, and despondency about his isolation from the scientific community, which viewed his sexual theories with suspicion and totally ignored *The Interpretation of Dreams* when it was published in 1900.

Insofar as he explicitly called the case history of Dora a "continuation of the dream book,"[17] Freud seems to authorize us to read the case as a symptomatic continuation of his ongoing self-analysis, as a fragment of the analysis of *his* case of hysteria. To view the text in this way is to see Freud as actively involved in a powerfully ambivalent countertransference. Resisting not only his desire for Dora but also, and more importantly in my view, his identification with her, Freud rejects as other and aberrant the feminine side of himself that he had embraced in the transferential relation with Fliess. He can accept his femininity, it seems, as a "passive" response (his term) to fantasized male superiority but not as an identification with a woman whose sexuality is pluralized through multiple bisexual impulses.

The consequent failure of the case in terms of Freud's self-analysis, the implicit subject of many of the essays in this volume, is thus crucially related to his "repudiation of femininity." And part of the fascination of the case for literary critics consists in the way Freud gives this repudiation a specifically narrative function. While admitting that his own text is fragmentary, full of detours, gaps, and omissions, he nevertheless insists on its difference from Dora's hysterically disjunctive and incoherent narrative. Thus the patient-analyst in attempting to cure himself is also involved in a kind of narrative cure, one intended to establish the dominance of a (male) discourse of scientific mastery (the privileged sphere of Fliess's expertise in the transference) over a duplicitous (female) tale of guilty fantasies and repressed desires. The productive failure of this therapeutic effort is a symptomatic narrative that invites us to read Dora as an overdetermined figure in Freud's unconscious, the name for those gaps in his self-knowledge whose intriguing hermeneutic, rhetorical, and psychosexual functions are teaching us to read anew.

Part Two

CLAIRE KAHANE

WHY DORA NOW?

It is by now self-evident that Freud has captured the imagination of those who engage in cultural inquiry. Like those creative writers whose narratives of the unconscious he appropriated for psychoanalysis, Freud knew the power of a good story to sustain the reader's interest. Although he wrote only a few case histories, they have figured as exemplary narratives in the history of psychoanalysis, each vividly dramatizing the process of his construction of the central paradigms of psychoanalytic theory. The "Fragment of an Analysis of a Case of Hysteria" has proven to be among the most elusive and fascinating of Freudian texts, for in spite of its having become the psychoanalytic model for the etiology of hysteria, it is a representation of the master's failure, of his inability to complete the story. Just as Freud could not let Dora go, at least imaginatively (as the text's history of delayed publication and added footnotes suggests),[18] so analysts have continually returned to the case to account for the difficulties that Freud encountered. The last several years in particular have seen an outpouring of interpretations of the case, coming more from literary critics, however, than from analysts. Why has this fragment commanded so much attention? Why do we now return to this failure of Freud's to complete his story of a sick girl in a sick milieu in *fin-de-siècle* Vienna? Why Dora now?

The answer to that question is as multidimensional as the reality that psychoanalysis has taught us to conceptualize, but if we look at the concerns that have predominated in discussions of the case, it is clear that *Dora* stands in the middle of a contemporary, interdisciplinary questioning of the relation between interpretation and sexual difference, a questioning initially fostered by Freud's writings and given new energy by recent feminist criticism. Certainly it is no accident that the Dora case occupies this intersection, for it was both the primary instance of the pitfalls of transference in interpretation and the only major case history that was the story of a woman. That conjunction was not coincidental: as many of the articles in this collection suggest, Freud's problem with transference was in great part a function of his relation to the story of a woman. The question that insists itself throughout psychoanalysis—What does a woman want?—was first answered by Freud in this case history, and it is not only the fragmentary and convoluted form of his answer, a hysterical narrative marked by transference, but its obsessively reiterated content that has provoked a return to Dora, to the place of sexual difference in the problematics of interpretation. What contemporary readings of Dora suggest is that, as brilliant as Freud was in constructing a narrative of Dora's desire, he essentially represented his own.

As we know, when Philip Bauer brought his eighteen-year-old daughter to see Freud, she had been suffering from recurrent aphonia, depression, and fits of coughing and had recently threatened suicide. Bauer told Freud that these symptoms derived from an incident that had occurred two years earlier, when the Bauers had joined their friends the K.'s at their vacation home by a lake in the Alps. Dora had accused Herr K. of propositioning her, had slapped his face and fled. Although since then she had urged her father to break off relations with the K.'s, Bauer, assured by his friend that Dora's tale was a fantasy, the result of a mind overstimulated by erotic books, asked Freud to "bring her to reason."

While Philip Bauer's story characterized Dora as a sexually disturbed adolescent girl subject to delusions, the story that emerges from

Freud's text is a melodrama of sexual politics riddled with illness and infidelity. Dora's father, engaged in an affair with Frau K., hands Dora over to Herr K. in return for his complicity, and although for many years Dora herself has raised no objections, even suppressing a sexual advance by Herr K. when she was fourteen, in the crucial scene at the lake, Dora refuses to be any longer a passive object in the circle of exchange. When her father hands her over to Freud to be made compliant, Freud, recognizing his motives, seems to refuse a complicit part and, instead, confirms Dora's perceptions. Yet Dora does have hysterical symptoms, and since, according to Freud's theory, hysterical symptoms are compromise formations that literally express repressed sexual wishes, Dora must have a secret, an unconscious desire. How does he determine what it is?

Since hysterics suffered from gaps in their memories, holes in their stories—the sign of repression—Freud's aim was to fill those gaps. Listening closely to the patient's communications—words, gestures, tone—Freud suggested meanings of which the patient was unaware, meanings which, extended to the symptoms, made of them signifiers—i.e. coded representations, that, when understood, formed part of a coherent narrative. When his patients came into possession of their own stories, Freud believed, they would not have to speak across the body. Yet Freud neglected to ask how a woman comes into possession of her own story, becomes a subject, when even narrative convention assigns her the place of an object of desire. How does an object tell a story? If, as hysteria disclosed, a story is told in symptoms, reading symptoms is not an easy or straightforward task. Symptoms are overdetermined just as language is. How does Freud choose from among the various potenital meanings an interpretation that will turn a fragmentary narrative into a coherent story?

From his own self-analysis as well as from his clinical work with hysterics—a conjunction that was not merely fortuitous, as Charles Bernheimer notes in part one of this introduction—Freud had derived a bold theory of psychic development impelled by sexual drives and culminating in the Oedipus complex. Although he would later revise its structure, at the time of the Dora case Freud's Oedipus complex is a simple set of relations in which the child desires the parent of the opposite sex and feels hostility for the same-sexed parent. In spite of his simultaneous belief in an innate bisexual disposition, Freud assumed a natural heterosexual attraction and saw his task as the liberation into consciousness of that natural desire, which, when repressed, resulted in hysterical symptoms. Thus, after imagining both Herr K.'s erection and Dora's arousal in her tale of his first sudden embrace, Freud concludes that Dora unconsciously desires the virile—and in his eyes entirely prepossessing—Herr K., a desire deriving from her infantile love for her father.

Although Freud continually presses Dora to admit her desire and accept this suitor chosen by her father, as several readers have observed,[19] it is not surprising that Dora resists the particularly sordid version of this nineteenth-century plot. What is surprising is Freud's blindness to a different story suggested by the material he restricts to the margins of his central narrative. Dora is not only attracted to her father but also identifies with him; she feels not only rivalry with the woman who is her father's love object but sexual desire. As Freud himself tells us, her love for Frau K. is the deepest unconscious current in her psychic life. Although he does not alter his basic plot, in the footnotes and digressions Freud suggests a fluidity of psychic identifications, of aim and object, that undermines his insistence on Dora's natural desire for the phallic male. Indeed, one can argue that it is that very fluidity, that psychic bisexuality that he elsewhere affirmed,[20] that allows Freud to interpret Dora's communications by means of his own associations, to read hysterical discourse by experiencing its source within himself. What Dora revealed was that sexual difference was a psychological problematic rather than a natural fact, that it existed within the individual psyche as well as between men and women in culture. Am I a man? Am I a woman? How is sexual identity assumed? How represented? These are the hysterical questions as Freud developed them out of the matrix of psychic bisexuality, as well as the central questions of psychoanalysis. Hysteria was thus the bedrock of psychoanalytic theory, and indeed, *Dora* in particular was meant to provide the ground for Freud's theoretical flights in *The Interpretation of Dreams.* As the history of its interpretations suggests, however, the text of *Dora,* like the protean fictions of hysteria, proved to be shifting sand. Not only did it reveal the terms "masculine" and "feminine" to be unmoored in the psychic life of hysterics, but the place of the analyst was opened to as much uncertainty as that of the analysand.

It is not surprising, then, that contemporary readers concerned with the problems of sexual difference in interpretation have been attracted to this elusive text. To be sure, among psychoanalysts the Dora case had always served as an example of the obstacles to interpretation, but the issue of sexual difference was scarcely considered. The first major case history that Freud recorded, *Dora* had impelled Freud, as it has subsequent analysts, to consider the reasons for his failure. Freud's conclusion, that its "great defect" was his inability to master the transference, led to a milestone in the history of psychoanalysis: the first elaboration of the role of transference, the patient's projection of a prior significant relation onto the relation with the analyst. Yet, as later analysts pointed out, Freud's remarks reveal only a very partial awareness of its extent.[21] More significantly for modern readers, never did he question the validity of his interpretation, or indicate an awareness of countertransference, the reciprocal process whereby the analyst's own wishes and fears are provoked by the patient. If Freud recognized that he had replaced both Dora's father and Herr K. in her imagination, he seemed not to question her place in his unconscious life and its effects on his interpretation.

In his 1951 article, "Intervention on the Transference," Jacques Lacan first described the relation between transference and countertransference as a dialectical process in which both patient and analyst are implicated: transference is a response to the analyst's countertransference, Lacan argues, a knife that cuts both ways. Because Freud was blind to the countertransference, based on his identification with a virile image of Herr K., he could not bring Dora out of her negative transference to a recognition of her desire. Although Lacan initiated a critique of countertransference in the Dora case that explicitly touched on Freud's unconscious attachment to a virile self-image and its consequences on his reading of Dora, because his article remained untranslated until recently, it had little effect on his American contemporaries. Thus, for example, when Felix Deutsch wrote his famous "Footnote to Freud's 'Fragment of an Analysis of a Case of Hysteria' " (1957), he did not question Freud's interpretative strategies but rather applauded his foresight, confirming it with additional facts about Dora's later life: her continued conversion symptoms, her hatred and distrust of men, and her eventual death from colonic cancer. Moreover, Deutsch first put into circulation a characterization of Dora, reported by a colleague, as "one of the most repulsive hysterics he had ever met," thus supporting the unself-conscious countertransferential image of the hysterical woman that still haunts psychoanalytic literature.

While Deutsch hoped that his footnote would stimulate a reappraisal of the process of conversion, subsequent psychoanalytic readings of the case were directed instead to Freud's own distortions or omissions, which had caused Dora to break off the treatment. Speaking of the case in 1961, Erik Erikson focused on the concerns of adolescent ego development that were absent from Freud's interpretation. Erikson located an essential problem in Freud's concept of "reality" and, reconceptualizing "reality" as "actuality," as what the ego verifies through action, argued that while Freud's genetic explanation of Dora's symptoms might be "true," another kind of truth, "historical truth," was a primary adolescent concern that Freud neglected. The actuality of Dora's history, her experience of multiple infidelities at a time when she needed to find fidelity, to have her assessment of circumstances verified, as well as the pervasive historical obstacles to acquiring a positive identity that confronted women of the time, led Dora to an identity as patient.

Erikson's reading of the case in terms of adaptive ego needs provoked other reconsiderations of Freud's Dora, but the question he had asked, What was it that Dora wanted from Freud?—the question of transference—has shifted over the last decade to the question of countertransference, What did Freud want from Dora? The most radical reconsiderations of that question have come from outside the psychoanalytic establishment, and, in recent years, particularly from feminist literary critics. For the feminist project that took shape in the late 1960s was to reexamine the cultural assumptions about femininity and female desire and to describe how those assumptions contributed to the circumscription of women. The Dora case is a particularly rich gift to this project: a paradigmatic text of patriarchal assumptions about female desire that still carry cultural authority and a vivid record of the construction of those assumptions as they emerge from the desire of the interpreter. Even more provocatively, the traces of Dora's story that form a subtext to Freud's oedipal narrative and continually disrupt it suggest an alternative preoedipal narrative that many feminists are reinscribing.

Paradoxically, the case could not reveal its value without the Freudian legacy, without an awareness of the processes of psychic transformations that Freud first described and that contemporary psychoanalysis continues to develop. Although early feminist readings of the case saw only Freud's misogyny, it is too easy and ultimately unproductive, as one critic in this collection remarks, to point simply to Dora's victimization by Freud's overarching interpretations, to see Dora only as a resistant heroine. Felix Deutsch's description of her unhappiness and morbid anxiety cannot be readily accommodated to a vision of her victorious heroinism. But by closely attending to the details of the text, a feminist psychoanalytic reading can open the case to the complex interweaving of fact and fantasy that comprises sexual politics both in the case and in the culture and that inevitably informs interpretation.

It seems particularly relevant that one of the most influential essays to reopen the Dora case in the last decade, Steven Marcus' "Freud and Dora: Story, History, Case History," drew this text out of the clinical discourse of psychoanalysis by treating it as a masterpiece of modernist fiction. Since both modernist fiction and hysterical narratives deny the possibility of any access to truth, since both are expressions of that perpetual displacement of meaning that contemporary critical theory attributes to discourse itself, Freud's narrative was ripe for an incisive literary analysis. Already in 1962, Philip Rieff had emphasized in his introduction to the Collier paperback edition the literary nature of the case history as a genre. In developing this new form, Rieff pointed out, Freud had introduced a new mode of historical writing. Its multiple analytical perspectives are analogous to the modernist effort to break linear narrative with its single chain of cause and effect. Extending Rieff's suggestion, Marcus traces Freud's formal innovations and multidimensional representations, but more importantly for feminist criticism, he shows how Freud rather than Dora ultimately becomes the central character, an unreliable narrator relentlessly pursuing his own demon of interpretation. In his often outrageous narration, Freud is more novelist than analyst, the reality he constructs as heterogeneous and ambiguous as a great fiction.

Regarding Freud as a novelist raises some provocative analogies, which Neil Hertz develops in "Dora's Secrets, Freud's Techniques." Comparing Freud's relation to Dora with that of Henry James and his character Maisie in *What Maisie Knew,* Hertz points out that when a middle-aged male novelist creates a female adolescent character, he writes out of an imaginative identification that we are accustomed to acknowledge in the genesis of a fiction but that is also operative in Freud's writing of a case history. In an elegant reading of Freud's defensive use of technique and technical language, Hertz demonstrates that Freud unconsciously identifies with his character: he is Dora, a young girl vulnerable to the authority of her elders, a hysteric whose discourse is full of holes.

In spite of Freud's insistence that a case history of hysteria must reflect hysterical fragmentation, as both Marcus and Hertz indicate, Freud was obsessively disconcerted by the fragmentary form of his narrative, which linked him to Dora. Marcus notes the various ways in which Freud repeatedly returns to the problem of fragments: the treatment was broken off; Freud analyzes only certain issues; only a part of the relevant material is brought up; the case is an abridged record that omits the process of interpretation; it is a singular case and thus a fragment of the entire structure of hysteria; Freud's insight is fragmentary because of the impossibility of reconstructing the past; the case is a fragment of Freud's larger project of demonstrating the relation between dreams and hysteria and depends upon a knowledge of *The Interpretation of Dreams,* its pre-text.

Even though Freud had already posited an essential core of mystery in the unconscious beyond which analysis could not go, so that every case would be ultimately a fragment, in the Dora case he assumes that "if the work continued, we should no doubt have obtained the fullest possible enlightenment upon every particular of the case." The implications of this phantasmatic "no doubt" are touched upon by various readers. In "Representations of Patriarchy: Sexuality and Epistemology in Freud's Dora," Toril Moi takes up the issue of Freud's obsessive desire for complete knowledge to argue that fragmentary knowledge implied impotence for Freud, that castration anxiety dominated his epistemological quest for phallic omnipotence. Thus where gaps existed, as Freud himself confessed, he "restored what is missing," attempting to create a totality that defied his own insights. Like Hertz, Moi uncovers Freud's masculine protest against the implications of his own femininity.

In a complementary essay, "Enforcing Oedipus: Freud and Dora," Madelon Sprengnether, considering the preoedipal nurse–invalid structure of sexual relations that pervades Freud's text, traces the ways in which Freud's reasoning, especially his construction of a virile interpretation of Herr K.'s embrace of Dora and the fellatio fantasy that he attributes to her, serves as a defense against his own orality, passive desire, and femininity. Thus Freud took pains to distinguish himself from Dora's impotent and invalid father, while the virile Herr K. remained an unquestioned figure of identification.

Although Freud later recognized that Dora had linked him to Herr K. in the transference, the five authors of "Questioning the Unconscious: The Dora Archive" argue that he failed to acknowledge a more threatening transference with Frau K., a woman who is the object of homosexual love as well as a maternal object. If Frau K. is a significant love object for Dora, she must also be part of the transference. Questioning Freud's repression of this transference, they point to specific structural instances of textual repression and conclude that what Freud occults in Dora's history—the mother and her subsequent displacements—he also occults in the theory of the Oedipus complex, which exemplifies "the repression of the mother . . . at the root of Western civilization itself."

What these feminist readings agree upon is that, at least in the Dora case, Freud's interpretive strategies were critically determined by his inability to deal with the feminine and its relation to the mother. If, as Charles Bernheimer notes in the first part of this introduction, Freud was able to admit his femininity in his correspondence with Fliess, as the analyst-father of Dora, he participated in that "rebellious overcompensation of the male" that he himself identified. By repressing his own feminine engagement as well as the place of the mother in Dora's history, Freud's narrative of female desire was inevitably fragmented. Certainly the history of his writings on femininity bears witness to his difficulties, for Freud repeatedly stumbled on the question of what a woman wants, and although by 1931 he had acknowledged the duration and intensity of the preoedipal relation of girls to their mothers, as in the Dora case, that originary desire remained marginal to his theorizing.[22] In Freud's more inclusive oedipal narrative, the little girl is first a little boy, actively desiring her mother in the preoedipal period. When she recognizes her lack—the penis she must have to gain her mother's love—she turns with hostility from her mother, represses her inappropriately phallic desire, takes her father as love object, and is thrust into the feminine position. From this revised perspective, Dora's hysteria is still interpreted by analysts as a consequence of her inability to assume her oedipal heterosexual destiny. Thus, in "Dora Revisited," Karl Lewin takes up Freud's idea that the mother is the primary love object for both sexes to suggest that all women are virtual hysterics, that the conflicts of Dora are those of all girls growing up, craving their mothers and envying their fathers' primacy, but having to displace their "homosexual love."[23]

Although Lewin does not question the necessity of that displacement, feminist readings of Dora have used that same concept—that the mother is the daughter's primary love object—to very different ends. Maria Ramas, for example, in "Freud's Dora, Dora's Hysteria," also states that, insofar as Dora's symptoms disguised a wish, it was her preoedipal desire for the mother and the maternal body. But Ramas places that desire within the context of a pervasive patriarchal fantasy of sadomasochistic sexual relations in which the feminine position is fixed as masochistically submissive. Thus Ramas reads Dora's hysteria as a failed protest against the sadistic meaning of the phallus and heterosexual postoedipal femininity.

Although not a Lacanian reading, Ramas' exploration of the relation between Dora's history and her historical context is clearly indebted to the work of Jacques Lacan. Translated in the 1970s, Lacan's writings introduced American critics, and especially feminists, to the psychic effects of language and culture. Lacan's own reading of Dora, however, rejects the importance of a historical referent for sexual trauma in the same way that Freud had rejected the historical reality of seduction. Just as Lacan distinguishes between the penis as biological organ and the phallus as signifier, he distinguishes between the actual father, who is relatively insignificant, and the paternal metaphor, the name of the Father in the Symbolic order represented by language. Lacan's Father is thus the *figure* of a function that breaks the Imaginary relation between self and other-as-image-of-self. Although Lacan would have Freud-as-analyst become this Symbolic Father, and lead Dora, through a dialectical movement that transcends the Imaginary, to assume her place within the order of sexual difference, because Freud himself was caught up in an imaginary identification with Herr K., he was unable to bring Dora to a positive transference.

What Lacanian feminists have found liberating in this father-dominated narrative is Lacan's disclosure of sexual difference as a construction in culture rather than, as in Freud's more conservative moments, a natural fact that determines destiny. Thus Suzanne Gearhart's "The Scene of Psychoanalysis: The Unanswered Questions of Dora" accedes to Lacan's reading up to a point. Like Lacan, she reads the scene by the lake as the primal scene of the case, and like Lacan, she notes Dora's simultaneous identification with both Herr and Frau K. That identification, based on the capacity of the subject to identify with either male or female in the primal scene, enables Dora to interpret Herr K.'s remark—"I get nothing out of my wife"—as an expression of *his* deficiency. Thus Dora discovers the imaginary nature of Herr K. as virile object to which Freud is blind. Gearhart, however, questions Lacan's defense of Freud. Lacan had argued, she notes, that Freud's assumption of a natural heterosexual attraction against which Dora's homosexuality would appear disruptive is later modified by his concept of bisexuality, which would have allowed Freud to reach a positive transference. Introducing the criticism of Luce Irigaray, Gearhart points to references in Freud's later writings in which he continues to "fall back" on "natural prejudices" in the same way that he envisages for Dora a "natural" solution, a marriage to Herr K. Ultimately Gearhart undermines Lacan's dialectical schematization by insisting on the endless process of bisexual identification in which both Freud and Dora participate.

What is implicit in Gearhart's reading is the explicit subject of Jacqueline Rose's "Dora: Fragment of an Analysis," a Lacanian interrogation of the case as the problem of the feminine within psychoanalysis. Like Gearhart, Rose questions Freud's concept of the feminine as bound to an insupportable notion of reality. Rejecting both the naturalist response of feminists who would locate a preoedipal content to female sexuality in the original mother–daughter relation, as well as a "natural" penis envy to explain the girl's rejection of her mother, Rose insists that sexuality is a function of insatiable desire and that the concepts of transference and unconscious representation as developed by Lacan have collapsed the category of sexuality as content. Thus Rose argues we must relinquish the idea of a specific feminine discourse, of a content-laden femininity, and replace it with the idea that the feminine is a relation to discourse, a revelation of the site of impossibility.

While Rose reads *Dora* as a key text in the contemporary discourse on femininity, in "Keys to Dora," Jane Gallop, another Lacanian feminist, moves that discourse into the political domain. Reading hysteria as the woman's story, Gallop inserts herself into a previously published dialogue about hysteria between Hélène Cixous and Catherine Clément in order to move that story further into the symbolic circuit of exchange, into published discourse by and about women. Provocatively commenting on the terms of the debate in which they engage—is Dora heroine or victim? Does she contest or conserve?—Gallop opens Freud's text and theirs to ambiguities that disrupt both the limits of their positions and the familiar, family-enclosed drama of psychoanalysis. Gallop criticizes as phantasmatic the apolitical psychoanalytic thinking that would reduce socioeconomic questions to family matters between parents and children and shows how the figure of the governess/maid with whom both Freud and Dora identify is the locus of intrusion into the bourgeois family of economic inferiority and sexual exploitation. A figure of threatening alterity that both Freud and Dora would repress or expel, she must be acknowledged by both analyst and patient, Gallop insists, if psychoanalysis is to remain vital. Just as a recognition of the commercial exchange between analyst and patient helps to disrupt the transference-idealization of the analyst, so the Imaginary assimilation of servant-nurse to phallic mother that denies the barter of women must be ruptured by the Symbolic, by acknowledgment of the system of exchange in which all women are objects.

As we can see, these contemporary readings of Freud's *Dora* raise issues that extend far beyond the clinical category of hysteria. Although Freud's assertion that hysteria afflicted both men and women was a liberating gesture in the nineteenth century, contemporary feminists are reclaiming hysteria as the dis-ease of women in patriarchal culture. *Dora* is thus no longer read as merely a case history or a fragment of an analysis of hysteria but as an urtext in the history of woman, a fragment of an increasingly heightened critical debate about the meaning of sexual difference and its effects on the representations of feminine desire. Standing at the intersection of psychoanalysis and feminism, the case of Dora, newly reopened, has pushed psychoanalysis from the consulting room into an ideological arena where it must engage in a dialogue with feminism and thus recover its radical promise. "We are bringing them the plague," Freud had remarked of his lectures on psychoanalysis delivered in the United States. The essays in this collection demonstrate how restorative that unlikely gift can be.

Notes

1. Catherine Clément and Hélène Cixous, *La jeune née* (Paris: 10/18, 1975), p. 283.
2. J. M. Charcot, *Lectures on the Diseases of the Nervous System*, George Gigerson, tr. (London: New Sydenham Society, 1877), p. 37. Quoted in Ilza Veith, *Hysteria: The History of a Disease* (Chicago: University of Chicago Press, 1965), p. 232. My presentation here is substantially based on this fine scholarly study.
3. *Malleus Maleficarum*, Montague Summers, tr. and ed. (London: Pushkin Press, 1951), p. 43. Quoted in Veith, p. 63.
4. Clément and Cixous, p. 23.
5. See Michel Foucault, *Madness and Civilization: A History of Insanity in the Age of Reason*, Richard Howard, tr. (New York: Pantheon, 1967), p. 121.
6. Thomas Sydenham, *Médicine pratique* (Paris, 1784), p. 394. Quoted in Foucault, p. 125.
7. See Foucault, pp. 204–222.
8. My discussion of the Victorian hysteric is indebted to that of Alan Krohn,

Hysteria: The Elusive Neurosis (New York: International Universities Press, 1978), pp. 176–186.

9. Freud, *Standard Edition of the Complete Psychological Works of Sigmund Freud*, James Strachey, tr. and ed., 24 vols. (London: Hogarth Press; New York: Macmillan, 1953–1974). Hereinafter cited as *SE* with appropriate volume and page number.

10. Dianne Hunter, "Hysteria, Psychoanalysis, and Feminism: The Case of Anna O.," *Feminist Studies* (Fall 1983), 9(3):467–468, 476.

11. Steven Marcus, "Introductory Essay," in Sigmund Freud, *The Origins of Psychoanalysis: Letters to Wilhelm Fliess* (New York: Basic Books, 1954), p. ix.

12. For an interesting discussion of the role of prostitution in the male imagination of Freud's time and place, see Sander Gilman, "Freud and the Prostitute: Male Stereotypes of Female Sexuality in *fin-de-siècle* Vienna," *Journal of the American Academy of Psychoanalysis* (1981), 9:3.

13. Clément and Cixous, p. 276.

14. See Jeffrey Masson, *The Assault on Truth: Freud's Suppression of the Seduction Theory* (New York: Farrar, Strauss, and Giroux, 1984), and Milton Klein "Freud's Seduction Theory: Its Implications for Fantasy and Memory in Psychoanalytic Theory," *Bulletin of the Menninger Clinic* (May 1981), vol. 45, no. 3. Masson's personality and his flamboyantly ambivalent relation to the psychoanalytic establishment are the subject of two lively articles by Janet Malcolm (*The New Yorker*, December 5 and 12), forthcoming in book form under the title *In the Freud Archives*.

15. William Warner, *Singular Repetition: An Essay on Chance and the Person*, forthcoming.

16. *The Origins of Psychoanalysis*, p. 169. The subsequent quotation is on p. 318. Both the letters in which these statements appear are omitted from the selection of the Fliess correspondence published in volume 1 of the Standard Edition.

17. *The Origins of Psychoanalysis*, p. 326.

18. For a full discussion of the history of publication, see Steven Marcus' essay in this volume.

19. The nineteenth-century structure of narrative expectations that informs Freud's case history is pointed out by Madelon Sprengnether and Claire Kahane in their introduction to *The M/Other Tongue*, a collection of feminist-psychoanalytic essays edited by Sprengnether, Kahane, and Shirley Garner, forthcoming from Cornell University Press.

20. Freud's exposition of psychic bisexuality occurs most fully in "Three Essays on the Theory of Sexuality," *SE* 7:125–245.

21. See especially the article by Hyman Muslin and Merton Gill in the Bibliography.

22. See Freud, "Female Sexuality" (1931), *SE* 21:225–243; and "Femininity" (1933), *SE* 22:112–135.

23. Karl Lewin, "Dora Revisited," *Psychoanalytic Review* (1974), vol. 60.

Biographical Note: Dora's Family

Dora's real name was Ida Bauer. She was born in Vienna on November 1, 1882, of Bohemian Jewish ancestry. The Bauers, however, were assimilated Jews who considered themselves more German than Czech and did not practice any religion. Her father, Philip, was a wealthy textile manufacturer who, as we find out from the case history, was in poor health throughout Dora's childhood, suffering first from tuberculosis, then a detached retina, and finally complications due to syphilis (contracted before his marriage), of which Freud cured him six years before the onset of Dora's analysis. He died of tuberculosis in 1913. All accounts of Dora's mother, Käthe, who died of the same disease a year before her husband, confirm that she was, in Freud's phrase, afflicted with "housewife's psychosis." Her obsession with cleanliness was such that she insisted that shoes be removed before entering the Bauer apartment, which had to be avoided altogether on days of "thorough" cleaning, and that she kept some rooms, including the salon, locked at all times, retaining the sole key in her possession. Her elaborate washing compulsions led Felix Deutsch, an analyst who had two interviews with Ida in 1922, to comment that "[Ida] and her mother saw the dirt not only in their surroundings, but also on and within themselves" (see essay 1 in this book). Their fears, however, were not without justification since Philip Bauer did literally contaminate his wife, bringing the sexual dirt from the surroundings into his home.

Ida Bauer married in 1903, a year after her last visit to Freud. Her husband was an unsuccessful composer employed by her father, who once hired an entire orchestra just to provide his son-in-law with the pleasure of hearing his music performed. We learn from Felix Deutsch's report that the marriage, at least from her point of view, was intensely unhappy. Having suffered a serious head and ear injury during the war, which affected his sense of balance and may have impaired his memory, the husband was never in good health and died of a heart ailment in 1932. Ida herself died of colonic cancer in New York City in 1945 and was survived by her only child, a son.

The member of the Bauer family about whom the most is known is Ida's brother Otto, who was one of the principal leaders of the Austrian Socialist party between 1918 and 1934 and its chief theoretician and ideological proponent (see the two articles by Arnold Rogow in the Bibliography). In contrast to the harsh criticism she directed against her husband, son, and father, Dora, in talking to Deutsch, "recalled with great feeling how close she had always been to her brother," a closeness that seems to be confirmed by Otto's having called Deutsch to express his concern for his sister's health and his desire to discuss her condition in person with the doctor. To his political colleagues, however, Otto appeared to be a severe, reserved, enigmatic man who worked tirelessly, authoring six major books and numerous journalistic articles as well as participating in countless party meetings and parliamentary debates. He was a creature of fixed habits who had some of his mother's obsessional characteristics (although a cleanliness compulsion was not among them). In view of the family history, it is interesting to note that he did not marry until 1914, two years after the death of his mother, to whom Freud had supposed him particularly attached. Moreover, he married a woman ten years his senior and already the mother of three. This maternally derived attachment did not last, however, and, like his father before him, he turned to a younger woman, who remained his mistress from 1928 until his death in Paris ten years later.

1. A Footnote to Freud's "Fragment of an Analysis of a Case of Hysteria"

FELIX DEUTSCH, M.D.

In his biography of Freud, Ernest Jones refers to the well-known case of Dora and to her various hysterical somatic and mental symptoms. After stating that she never resumed her analysis of only eleven weeks' duration, he mentions that she "died a few years ago in New York."[1]

For several reasons this fact aroused my interest. What did she die from? Could Freud's intuition and penetrating interpretation of only two dreams really bring to light the personality structure of this unfortunate girl? If he was right, should not the course of her later life bear out Freud's views of the various motives for retaining her conversion symptoms? And last but not least, how much further advanced are we today in understanding the "leap from the mental into the physiological"?

My particular curiosity about Dora's later life would have met an insurmountable obstacle from the beginning during Freud's life because of his discretion. He wrote:

This essay was first published in *Psychoanalytic Quarterly* (1957), 26:159–167.

I have waited for four whole years since the end of the treatment, and have postponed publication till hearing that a change has taken place in the patient's life of such a character as allows me to suppose that her own interest in the occurrences and psychological events which are to be related here may now have grown faint. Needless to say, I have allowed no name to stand which could put a nonmedical reader upon the scent; and the publication of the case in a purely scientific and technical periodical should, further, afford a guarantee against unauthorized readers of this sort. Naturally I cannot prevent the patient herself from being pained if her own case history should accidentally fall into her hands. But she will learn nothing from it that she does not already know; and she may ask herself who besides her could discover from it that she is the subject of this paper.(*SE* 7–8; *C* 22–23)

Twenty-four years after Freud's treatment of Dora, an event took place that dispelled the anonymity of this case to another analyst without Freud's knowledge. In a footnote to the "Postscript" of "A Fragment of an Analysis of a Case of Hysteria," Freud wrote:

The problem of medical discretion which I have discussed in this preface does not touch the remaining case histories contained in this volume; for three of them were published with the express assent of the patients (or rather, as regards little Hans, with that of his father), while in the fourth case (that of Schreber) the subject of the analysis was not actually a person but a book produced by him. In Dora's case the secret was kept until this year. I had long been out of touch with her, but a short while ago I heard that she had recently fallen ill again from other causes, and had confided to her physician that she had been analyzed by me when she was a girl. This disclosure made it easy for my well-informed colleague to recognize her as the "Dora" of 1899. No fair judge of analytic therapy will make it a reproach that the three months' treatment she received at that time effected no more than the relief of her current conflict and was unable to give her protection against subsequent illnesses. (*SE* 7:13–14n; *C* 28*n*)[2]

Freud withheld the name of the consulting physician in agreement with him, since it might have led to the disclosure of the patient's identity. Now that Dora is no longer alive, it can be revealed, without transgressing the discretion that protected her anonymity, why the note in Jones' book about Dora's death aroused my special interest. The reason is that I am the physician who told Freud in 1922 of my encounter with Dora. It happened shortly after the presentation of my paper, "Some Reflections on the Formation of the Conversion Symptom," at the Seventh International Psychoanalytic Congress in Berlin, in September 1922, the last that Freud attended. I referred to some of the viewpoints raised in that paper and to the mysterious "leap from the mind to the soma" when I told Freud how my encounter with Dora took place and how I had *nolens volens* been let into the secret.

In the late fall of 1922, an otolaryngologist asked my opinion about a patient of his, a married woman, forty-two years old, who for some time had been bedridden with marked symptoms of Ménière's syndrome: tinnitus, decreased hearing in the right ear, dizziness, and sleeplessness because of continual noises in this ear. Since an examination of the inner ear, of the nervous system, as well as of the vascular system showed no pathology whatever, he inquired whether a psychiatric study of the patient, who behaved very "nervously," might perhaps explain her condition.

The interview began in the presence of her physician. Her husband left the room shortly after he had listened to her complaints and did not return. She started with a detailed description of the unbearable noises in her right ear and of dizziness when moving her head. She had always suffered from periodic attacks of migraine on the right side of her head. The patient then started a tirade about her husband's indifference toward her sufferings and how unfortunate her marital life had been. Now her only son had also begun to neglect her. He had recently finished college and had to decide whether he should continue with his studies. However, he often stayed out late at night and she suspected he had become interested in girls. She always waited, listening, until he came home. This led her to talk about her own frustrated love life and her frigidity. Another pregnancy had appeared to her to be impossible because she could not endure the labor pains.

Resentfully she expressed her conviction that her husband had been unfaithful to her, that she had considered divorce, but could not decide what to do. Tearfully she denounced men in general as selfish, demanding, and ungiving. That brought her back to her past. She recalled with great feeling how close she had always been to her brother, who had become the leader of a political party and who still visited whenever she needed him—in contrast to her father, who had been unfaithful even to her mother. She reproached her father for having once had an affair with a young married woman whom she, the patient, had befriended, and whose children had been for some time under her care when she was a young girl. The husband of this woman had then made sexual advances to her, which she had rejected.

This story sounded familiar to me. My surmise about the identity of the patient was soon confirmed. In the meantime, the otologist had left the room. The patient then began to chat in a flirtatious manner, inquiring whether I was an analyst and whether I knew Professor Freud. I asked her in turn whether she knew him and whether he had ever treated her. As if having waited for this cue, she quickly replied that she was the "Dora" case, adding that she had not seen a psychiatrist since her treatment with Freud. My familiarity with Freud's writings evidently created a very favorable transference situation.

She forgot to talk about her sickness, displaying great pride in having been written up as a famous case in psychiatric literature. Then she spoke of the failing health of her father, who now often seemed out of his mind. Her mother had recently been admitted to a sanitarium to be treated for tuberculosis. She suspected that her mother might have acquired the tuberculosis from her father, who, as she remembered, had this disease when he was a child. She apparently had forgotten her father's history of syphilis, which Freud mentioned and which he considered in general a constitutional predisposition and a "very relevant factor in the aetiology of the neuropathic constitution in children." She also expressed concern about her occasional colds and difficulties in breathing, as well as her coughing spells in the morning, which she thought were due to her excessive smoking during past years. As if wanting to make this more acceptable, she said her brother had the same habit, too.

When I asked her to leave the bed and to walk around, she walked with a slight limp of the right leg. Questioned about the limp, she could give no explanation. She had had it since childhood, but it was not always noticeable. Then she discussed Freud's interpretation of her two dreams and asked my opinion about it. When I ventured to connect her Ménière's syndrome with her relationship to her son and with her continual listening for his return from his nightly excursions, she appeared ready to accept it and asked for another consultation with me.

The next time I saw her she was out of bed and claimed that her "attacks" were over. The Ménière's symptoms had disappeared. Again she released a great amount of hostile feeling toward her husband, especially her disgust with marital life. She described her premenstrual pains and a vaginal discharge after menstruation. Then she talked mainly about her relationship to her mother, of her unhappy childhood because of her mother's exaggerated cleanliness, her annoying washing compulsions, and her lack of affection for her. Mother's only concern had been her own constipation, from which the patient herself now suffered. She finally spoke with pride about her brother's career, but she had little hope that her son would follow in his footsteps. When I left her, she thanked me eloquently and promised to call me if she should feel the need. I never heard from her again. Her brother called several times shortly after my contact with his sister, expressing his satisfaction with her speedy recovery. He was greatly concerned about her continual suffering and her discord with both her husband and their mother. He admitted it was difficult to get along with her because she distrusted people and attempted to turn them against each other. He wanted to see me at my office, but I declined in view of Dora's improvement.

One can easily understand that this experience made me want to compare the clinical picture of the patient with the one Freud had described in his brief analysis twenty-four years earlier when she was eighteen years old. It is striking that Dora's fate took the course Freud had predicted. He admitted that "the treatment of the case and consequently my insight into the complex of events composing it, remained fragmentary. There are therefore many questions to which I have no solution to offer, or in which I can only rely upon hints and conjectures" (*SE* 7–23*n*; *C* 38n). These considerations, however, did not alter his basic concept that "the majority of hysterical symptoms, when they have attained their full pitch of development, represent an imagined situation of sexual life." Unquestionably Dora's attitude toward marital life, her frigidity, and her disgust with heterosexuality bore out Freud's concept of displacement, which he described in these terms: "I can arrive at the following derivation for the feelings of disgust. Such feelings seem originally to be a reaction to the *smell* (and afterwards also to the *sight*) of excrement. But the genitals can act as a reminder of the excremental functions" (*SE* 7:31; *C* 47).

Freud corroborated this concept later in his "Notes Upon a Case of Obsessional Neurosis," referring to the patient as "a *renifleur*" (osphresiolagniac), being more susceptible to sensations of smell than most people. Freud adds in a footnote that the patient "in his childhood had been subject to strong coprophilic propensities. In this connection his *anal erotism* has already been noticed" (*SE* 10:247n.; italics added).

We may ask, apart from the senses of *smell, taste,* and *vision,* whether other propensities for the use of *sensory* perception were involved in the conversion process of Dora. Certainly the *auditory* apparatus played an important role in the Ménière's syndrome. In fact, Freud refers to Dora's dyspnoea as apparently conditioned by her listening as a child to the noises in her parents' bedroom, which had then adjoined her own. This "listening" was repeated in her alertness for the sound of her son's footsteps when he returned home at night after she suspected he had become interested in girls.

As for her sense of *touch,* she had showed its repression in her contact with Mr. K. when he embraced her and when she behaved as if she had not noticed the contact with his genitals. She could not deny the contact of her lips when Mr. K. kissed her, but she *defended* herself against the effect of this kiss by denying her own sexual excitement and her awareness of Mr. K.'s genitals, which she rejected with disgust.

We must remember that in 1894 Freud proposed the name "conversion" as a *defense,* when he arrived at the concept that "in hysteria the unbearable idea is rendered innocuous by the quantity of excitation attached to it being transmuted into some bodily form of expression" (*SE* 3:49). Even earlier, in collaboration with Breuer, he phrased it: "The increase of the sum of excitation takes place along sensory paths and its diminution along motor ones. . . . If, however, there is no reaction whatever to a psychical trauma, the memory of it retains the affect which it originally had." That still holds true today.

Many years went by during which Dora's ego continued in dire need of warding off her feelings of guilt. We learn that she tried to achieve it by an identification with her mother, who suffered from a "housewife's psychosis" consisting of obsessional washing and other kinds of excessive cleanliness. Dora resembled her not only physically but also in this respect. She and her mother saw the dirt not only in their surroundings, but also on and within themselves. Both suffered from genital discharges at the time Freud treated Dora, as well as when I saw her.

It is striking that the dragging of her foot, which Freud had observed when the patient was a girl of eighteen, should have persisted twenty-five years. Freud stated that "a symptom of this kind can only arise when it has an infantile prototype" (*SE* 7:103; *C* 124). Dora had once twisted this foot when she was a child, slipping on a step as she was going downstairs. The foot had swelled and was bandaged, and she was kept in bed some weeks. It appears that such a symptom may persist through life, whenever there is a need to use it for the somatic expression of displeasure. Freud always adhered to "the concept of the biological rules" and considered displeasure "as being stored up for their protection. The somatic compliance, organically predetermined, paves the way for the discharge of an unconscious excitation."

The truth of Freud's statement that "it appears to be far more difficult to create a fresh conversion than to form paths of association between a new thought which is in need of discharge and the old one which is no longer in need of it" (*SE* 7:53; *C* 71) cannot be overemphasized. The somewhat fatalistic conclusion that one might draw from Dora's personality, which twenty-five years later was manifested as Freud had seen and foreseen it, is that she could not escape her destiny. However, this statement needs some qualification. Freud himself states very clearly that he had not published the case "to put the value of psychoanalytic therapy in its true light" and that the briefness of the treatment (which hardly lasted three months) was only one of the reasons that prevented a longer lasting improvement of Dora's condition (*SE* 7:115; *C* 137). Even if Freud had already made at that time his discoveries about transference neurosis and working through, Dora could not have benefited from them because she broke off the treatment unexpectedly as "an unmistakable act of vengeance on her part. Her purpose of self-injury also profited by this action" (*SE* 7:109; *C* 131).

More than thirty years have elapsed since my visit at Dora's sickbed. I would never have known anything more had Dr. Jones' note of her death in New York not helped me obtain further information concerning her later life. From my informant I learned the additional pertinent facts about the fate of Dora and of her family recorded here.

Her son brought her from France to the United States. Contrary to her expectations, he succeeded in life as a renowned musician. She clung to him with the same reproachful demands she made on her husband, who had died of a coronary disease—slighted and tortured by her almost paranoid behavior. Strangely enough, he had preferred to die, as my informant put it, rather than to divorce her. Without question, only a man of this type could have been chosen by Dora for a husband. At the time of her analytic treatment she had stated unequivocally: "Men are all so detestable that I would rather not marry. This is my revenge." Thus her marriage had served only to cover up her distaste of men.

Both she and her husband had been driven out of Vienna during World War II and emigrated initially to France. Before that she had been repeatedly treated for her well-known attacks of hemicranial migraine, coughing spells, and hoarseness, which Freud had analytically interpreted when she was eighteen years old.

In the early 1930s, after her father's death, she began to suffer from palpitations of the heart, which were thought to be caused by her excessive smoking. She reacted to these sensations with anxiety attacks and fear of death. This ailment kept everyone in her environment in continual alarm, and she utilized it to play off friends and relatives against each other. Her brother, also a chain-smoker, died much later from coronary disease in Paris, where he had escaped under the most adventurous circumstances. He was buried there with the highest honors.

Dora's mother died of turberculosis in a sanitarium. I learned from my informant that she had had the disease in her youth. She worked herself to death by her never-ending, daily cleaning compulsion—a task that nobody else could fulfill to her satisfaction. Dora followed in her footsteps, but directed the compulsion mainly to her own body. As her vaginal discharge persisted, she had several minor gynecological operations. The inability to "clean out her bowels," her constipation, remained a problem to the end of her life. Being accustomed to this trouble with her bowels, she apparently treated it as a familiar symptom until it became more than a conversion symptom. Her death from a cancer of the colon, which was diagnosed too late for a successful operation, seemed a blessing to those who were close to her. She had been, as my informant phrased it, "one of the most repulsive hysterics" he had ever met.

The additional facts about Dora presented here are no more than a footnote to Freud's postscript. I hope that presenting them now may stimulate reappraisal and discussion of the degree to which the concept of the process of conversion, in the sense Freud used it, is still valid, or in what respects it differs from our present-day comprehension of it.

Notes

1. Ernest Jones, *The Life and Work of Sigmund Freud*, vol. 2 (London: Hogarth Press, 1955), p. 289.
2. This footnote is actually to be found in the "Prefatory Remarks" to the *Dora* case—Editors' note.

2. Reality and Actuality: An Address

ERIK H. ERIKSON

One of the stories of Freud's preanalytic years that assumes a mythological quality in our training is the event at one of Charcot's evening receptions when the master during a bit of shop talk about hysteria in women "suddenly broke out with great animation: *Mais, dans des cas pareils c'est toujours la chose génitale, toujours . . . toujours . . . toujours.'* . . . I know that for a moment I was almost paralysed with amazement and said to myself: 'Well, but if he knows that, why does he never say so?' But the impression was soon forgotten; brain anatomy . . . absorbed all my interest" ("On the History of the Psychoanalytic Movement," *SE* 14:14).

Since then we have come full cycle. Freud's elucidation of "*la chose génitale*" has revolutionized psychology, and this Association has become the representative of that revolution in this country. Heirs of radical innovation, however, carry a double burden: they must do to-

This essay represents approximately half of the text of a talk delivered before the plenary session of the American Psychoanalytic Association in New York, 1961. It was first published in the *Journal of the American Psychoanalytic Association* (1962), 10:451–74. A revised version is printed as chapter 5 of the author's *Insight and Responsibility* (New York: Norton, 1964).

gether what the founder did in lonely years and also strive to keep ahead of the habituations that result from success. They may well, at intervals, ask themselves what they have come to know and what they on occasion say with "much animation," without pursuing it with the momentum of discovery.

One such item, I submit, is our knowledge of human strength. We have all heard psychoanalysts (including ourselves), in private conversations or in unguarded moments of clinical discussion, describe with wonder the evidences for some patient's regained health. Such evidences often seem hard to classify because they appear to have resulted from unexpected encounters "in the outside world" and from opportunities beyond our theoretical anticipations. During a recent discussion in a small circle, a great teacher in our field made the observation that children who feel loved become more beautiful. What it is, however, that transforms the whole appearance and pervades the very functioning of persons—that we have as yet no systematic way of studying. Maybe a method called analytic cannot and need not encompass such phenomena; but perhaps we tend to shy away from the manifestations of the human spirit, which theology and esthetics have monopolized for so long. A similar dilemma was circumscribed by W. H. Auden in a book review in which he pointed out how difficult it is for the psychoanalyst to conceptualize *deeds* as well as *behavior,* that is (to paraphrase him), to differentiate between individual action that makes a memorable difference in the shared lives of many and such stereotyped behavior as can be studied in clinical isolation.[1] Is this an essential limitation of psychoanalysis? Can we conceptualize man only in acute inner conflict, that is to say, retreating from or preparing for those moments when "his virtues . . . go forth of him"?

I frankly do not know whether today I will confirm such limitations or point beyond them as I discuss from a number of angles my impression that our often half-hearted and ambiguous conceptualization of reality has resulted in a failure to account for important features of adaptive and productive action and their relation to the major phenomena of ego strength.

What do we mean when we speak of the recognition of and the adjustment to reality? Hartmann has formulated the reality principle as the "tendency to take into account in an adaptive way . . . whatever we consider the *real features* of an object or situation,"[2] and the psychoanalytic usage of the term *reality* was quite recently stated again by Loewald as "the world of things *really existing* in the outer world."[3] Freud's criteria of reality are (as Hartmann has not uncritically pointed out) "the criteria of science, or more correctly, those that find their clearest expression in science . . . which accepts as 'objective' what is *verifiable by certain methods*" (Hartmann, "Notes," italics added). The psychoanalytic method, then, by its very design attempts to further man's adjustment by helping him to perceive facts and motives "as they are," that is, as they appear to the rational eye. Yet, Hartmann has also clarified the limited applicability of such rationalism to human adaptation[4]—a rationalism that would expose man to the dilemma of the centipede that found itself completely immobilized because it had been asked to watch carefully which of its feet it was going to put forward next. If Hartmann's approach to these matters develops from the consideration of thought, attention, and judgment to that of action, he follows faithfully, although he expands it firmly, the course of psychoanalytic preoccupation with reality. But this thinking harbors such terms as "acting *in regard* to reality," "action vis-à-vis reality," and "*acting in the outer world.*"[5] Maybe our habitual reference to man's environment as an "*outer world*" attests, more than any single term, to the fact that the world of action is still foreign territory to our theory. This term, more than any other, represents the Cartesian straitjacket that we have imposed on our model of man, who in some of our writings seems to be most himself when reflecting horizontally—like a supine baby or a reclining patient, or like Descartes, taking to his bed to cogitate on the extensive world. But, as I said, we know better than that in our daily clinical dealings, and I propose to discuss what we do know by separating from our concept of *reality* one of its more obscure implications, namely, *actuality,* the world verified only in the ego's immediate immersion in action. The German word *Wirklichkeit,* often implied in Freud's use of the word *Realität,* does combine *Wirkung,* that is, activity and efficacy, with reality.[6]

But before attempting to redefine actuality in ego terms, let me in our traditional manner illustrate its clinical relevance by discussing a question we have all asked ourselves as students: what *was* it that Dora wanted from Freud?

When we use Freud's work for the elucidation of what we are groping to say, it is for one very practical reason: all of us know the material by heart. Beyond this, we always find in Freud's writings parenthetical data worthy of the attention of generations to come. We must assume, of course, that Freud selected and disguised the clinical data he published, thus rendering reinterpretations hazardous. Yet, the repeated study of Freud's case reports strengthens the impression that we are dealing with creations of a high degree of psychological relevance and equivalence even in matters of peripheral concern to the author. Freud concludes his report on the treatment of Dora with an admission as frank as it is rare in professional publications: "I do not know what kind of help she wanted from me" (*SE* 7:122; *C* 144).

Dora, you will remember, had interrupted the treatment after only three months but had come back a year later (she was twenty years old then) "to finish her story and ask for help once more." But what she told him then did not please Freud. She had in the interval confronted her family with certain irresponsible acts previously denied by them, and she had forced them to admit their pretenses and their secrets. Freud considered this forced confrontation an act of revenge not compatible with the kind of insight that he had tried to convey to the patient through the analysis of her symptoms. The interview convinced him that "she was not in earnest over her request" for more help, and he sent her away. His displeasure he expressed in the assurance—apparently not solicited by the patient—that he was willing "to forgive her for having deprived [him] of the satisfaction of affording her a far more radical cure for her troubles" (*SE* 7:122; *C* 144). Since Dora was intelligent, however, the judgment that she was "not in earnest" suggested insincerity on her part. And, indeed, Felix Deutsch, who was consulted by Dora in her late middle age, gives an unfavorable picture of her fully developed character—as unfavorable as may be seen in clinical annals (see essay 1). Yet, in Freud's original description of the girl, Dora appeared "in the first bloom of youth—a girl of intelligent and engaging looks." If "an alteration in her character" indeed became one of the permanent features of her illness, one cannot help feeling that Dora was, as it were, confirmed in such change by the discontinuance of her treatment.

The description of Freud's fragmentary work with Dora has become the classical analysis of the structure and the genesis of a hysteria. It is clear from his description that Freud's original way of working and reporting was determined by his first professional identity as a physiological investigator: his clinical method was conceived as an analogy to clean and exact laboratory work. It focused on the "intimate structure of a neurotic disorder"—a structure that was really a reconstruction of its genesis and a search for the energies, the "quantities of excitation," that had been "transmuted" into the presenting symptoms, according to the dominant physicalistic configurations of his era.[7]

As to the unbearable excitations "transmuted" into Dora's symptoms, may it suffice to remind you of the two traumatic sexual approaches made to the girl by a Mr. K., a married man who kissed her once when she was fourteen under circumstances indicating that he had set the scene for a more thorough seduction, and who propositioned her quite unequivocally at an outing by an alpine lake when she was sixteen. She had rebuked the man; but the sensations, affects, and ideas aroused on these two occasions were translated into the symptom language of hysteria, which was then decoded by Freud. But how clinically alive and concrete is his quesion as to what more, or what else, Dora had a right to expect of him? He could not see, Freud relates, how it could have helped her if he "had acted a part . . . and shown a warm personal interest in her." No patient's demands, then, were to make him dissimulate his integrity as an investigator and his commitment to the genetic kind of truth: they were *his* criteria of the respect due to a patient. But if in the patient's inability to live up to his kind of truth Freud primarily saw repressed instinctual strivings at work, he certainly also noted that Dora, too, was in search of some kind of truth. He was puzzled by the fact that the patient was "almost beside herself at the idea of its being supposed that she had merely fancied" the conditions which had made her sick and that she kept "anxiously trying to make sure whether I was being quite straightforward with her." Let us remember here that Dora's father had asked Freud "to bring her to reason." Freud was to make his daughter let go of the subject of her seduction by Mr. K. The father had good reason for this wish, for Mr. K.'s wife was his own mistress, and he seemed willing to ignore Mr. K.'s indiscretions if he only remained unchallenged in his own. It was, therefore, highly inconvenient that Dora should insist on becoming morbid over her role as an object of erotic barter.

I wonder how many of us can follow today without protest Freud's assertion that a healthy girl of fourteen would, under such circumstances, have considered Mr. K.'s advances "neither tactless nor offensive." The nature and severity of Dora's pathological reaction make her the classical hysteric of her case history; but her motivation for falling ill, and her lack of motivation for getting well, today seem to call for developmental considerations. Let me pursue some of these.

Freud's report indicates that Dora was concerned with the historical truth as known to others, while her doctor insisted on the genetic truth behind her own symptoms. At the same time she wanted her doctor to be "truthful" in the therapeutic relation, that is, to keep faith with her on her terms rather than on those of her father or seducer. That her doctor did keep faith with her in terms of his investigative ethos she probably appreciated up to a point; after all, she did come back. But why then confront him with the fact that she had confronted her parents with the historical truth?

This act may impress some of us even today as "acting out." With Freud, we may predict that the patient would gain a permanent relief from her symptoms only by an ever better understanding of her own unconscious, an understanding that would eventually permit her to adjust to "outer reality," meaning to what cannot be helped. Strictly speaking, however, we could expect such utilization of insight only from a "mature ego," and Dora's neurosis was rooted in the crisis of adolescence.[8] The question arises whether today we would consider the patient's emphasis on the historical truth a mere matter of resistance to the genetic one or whether we would discern in it also an adaptive pattern genuine for her stage of life and challenged by her circumstances.

The introduction into psychoanalytic thinking of an adaptive point of view has brought to the fore some neglected features of the ego's total task of synthesis and adaptation.[9] Of all the aspects of a person's experience that are *acutely relevant to the ego's functioning* at a given time, we have learned to understand best the role of the *past* which is acutely relevant insofar as it makes effective claims on the present for repetition or remembrance; we have paid less attention to the *future*, acute insofar as it is anticipated and, in fact, created in immediate choice. The demands of *drives*, recognizable in acute needs and defenses are well studied; not so the role of developing *capacities*, which add new modes to the ego's power of adaptation. We have studied man's "*inner world*" with unprecedented devotion; yet we assign acutely decisive encounters, opportunities, and challenges to a nebulous "outer reality." One thing is immediately clear: each stage of development has its own acuteness and actualness, because a stage is a new configuration of past and future, a new combination of drive and defense, a new set of capacities fit for a new setting of tasks and opportunities, a new and wider radius of significant encounters. Our question, then, concerns the possibility that at each stage what appears to us as "acting out" may contain an element of action, that is, an adaptive if immature reaching out for the mutual verification by which the ego lives, and that, in *young adulthood*, the pursuit of factual or historical truth may be of acute relevance to the ego's adaptive strength.

There are, of course, many ways in which a young person may express a sudden preoccupation with truth—at first perverse and obsessive, changeable and pretentious, and altogether defensive in Anna Freud's sense,[10] but gradually taking hold of relevant issues and productive commitments. He may come to have a personal stake in the accuracy, veracity, and authenticity, in the fairness, genuineness, and reliability of persons, of methods, and of ideas. I have elsewhere postulated the quality of *Fidelity* as the essence of all those preoccupations.[11] As powerful new drives must find sanctioned expression or be kept in abeyance, and as regressive pulls must be resisted, it is a prime necessity for the ego that the capacity to pledge and receive fidelity emerge and mature during this period—even as societies, for the sake of their rejuvenation, must receive from their youth, by way of all manner of "confirmations," the pledge of particular fidelities in the form of ideological commitment.

Piaget and Inhelder, who have studied the thought process of adolescents by facing them with certain experimental tasks, have recognized in adolescence the ripening of a mode of thinking both hypothetical and deductive.[12] That is, the adolescent, before beginning to manipulate the material at hand, as the preadolescent would with little hesitation, waits and hypothesizes on the possible results, even as after the experiment he lingers and tries to fathom the truth behind the known results. This capacity forms, I think, a basis for the development, in later adolescence, of the *historical perspective,* which makes room not only for an imaginative speculation as to all that could have happened in the past but also for a deepening concern with the narrowing down of vast possibilities to a few tantalizing alternatives, often resolved only by a "totalistic" search for single causes. Youth is, at the same time, preoccupied with the danger of hopeless determination, be it by irreversible childhood identifications or otherwise "stacked" conditions, and yet also with the question of freedom in many urgent forms. Where a sense of restraint prevails, the quest for its causes becomes an ideological one, defying a merely intellectual approach. Thus, what we would call a genetic explanation to youth easily becomes a fatalistic one. Patients such as Dora, therefore, may insist that the genetic meaning of their sickness find recognition within an assessment of the historical truth, which at the same time clarifies the determination of what has become irreversible and promises the freedom of what is yet undetermined.

The employment of the particular cognitive gains of any stage of life is thus not just a matter of exercising intelligence: for these gains are part of a new pattern of verification that pervades a person's whole being. We know in pathology that certain forms of psychopathic evasion and psychotic denial depend for their full development on the fate of the established historical perspective in adolescence: only he who comprehends something of the nature of factual and historical truth can attempt to circumvent or deny it.

To return once more to Dora: if fidelity is a central concern of young adulthood, then her case appears to be a classical example of fatefully perverted fidelity. A glance back at her history will remind us that her family had exposed her to multiple sexual *infidelity,* while all concerned—father and mother, Mr. K. and Mrs. K.—tried to compensate for all their pervading *perfidy* by making Dora their *confidante*, each burdening her (not without her perverse provocation, to be sure) with half-truths that were clearly unmanageable for an adolescent. It is interesting to note that the middle-aged Dora, according to Felix Deutsch's report, was still obsessed with infidelities—her father's, her husband's, and her son's—and still turned everybody against everybody else (see essay 1). Lest it appear that I agree with those Victorian critics to whom Dora seemed only a case illustrating typical Viennese and sexual infidelity, however, I must add that other and equally malignant forms of fidelity-frustration pervade late adolescent case histories in other societies and periods.

If fidelity, then, emerges against the background of diverse historical perspectives, *identity*—as I had an opportunity to report to you a few years ago—must prove itself against sometimes confusing role demands.[13] As a *woman*, Dora did not have a chance. A vital identity fragment in her young life was that of the *woman intellectual*, which had been encouraged by her father's delight in her precocious intelligence but discouraged by her brother's superior example as favored by the times: she was absorbed in such evening education as was then accessible to a young woman of her class. The negative identity of the "*déclassée*" *woman* (so prominent in her era) she tried to ward off with her sickness: remember that Mr. K., at the lake, had tried to seduce her with the same argument which, as she happened to know, had previously been successful with a domestic. She may well have sought in Mrs. K., whom Freud recognized primarily as an object of Dora's ambivalent homosexual love, that mentor who helps the young to overcome unusable identifications with the parent of the same sex; Dora read books with Mrs. K. and took care of her children. But, alas, there was no escape from her mother's "*housewife's psychosis*," which Dora blended with her own then fully acquired *patient identity*. Felix Deutsch reports that the middle-age Dora, "chatting in a flirtatious manner . . . forgot . . . about her sickness, displaying great pride in having been written up as a famous case" (see essay 1). To be a famous, if uncured, patient had become for this woman one lasting positive identity element; in this she kept faith with Freud. We know today that if patienthood is permitted to become a young patient's most meaningful circumstance, his identity formation may seize on it as a central and lasting theme.

This brings us, finally, to the question of the devlopmental aspects of the therapeutic relationshp itself. At the time, Freud was becoming aware of the singular power of transference, and he pursued this in his evidence. Today we know that this most elemental tie always is complemented by the patient's relation to the analyst as a "new person."[14] Young patients in particular appoint and invest the therapist with the role of mentor, although he may strenuously resist expressing what he stands for. This does not obligate him, of course, to "play a part," as Freud so firmly refused to do. True mentorship, far from being a showy form of emotional sympathy, is part of a discipline of outlook and method. But the psychotherapist must recognize what role he is, in fact, playing in what we are here trying to circumscribe as the actuality of a young person.

In summary, it is probable that Dora needed to act as she did not only in order to vent the childish rage of one victimized but also in order to set straight the historical past so that she could envisage a sexual and social future of her choice, call infidelities by their name before she could commit herself to her own kind of fidelity, and establish the coordinates of her identity as a young woman of her class and time, before she could utilize more insight into her inner realities.

Beyond the case of Dora, however, we face here a problem of general therapeutic urgency: some mixture of *"acting out"* and of *age-specific action* is to be expected of any patient of whatever age; and all patients reach a point in treatment when the recovering ego may need to test its untrained or long-inhibited wings of action. In the analysis of children, we honor this to some extent; but in some excessively prolonged treaments of patients of all ages, we sometimes miss that critical moment, while remaining adamant in our pursuit of totally cleansing the patient of all "resistance to reality." Is it not possible that such habitual persistence obscures from us much of the ego's relation to action, and this under the very conditions that would make observation possible on clinical homeground?

You may wonder whether Dora's dreams, the focus of Freud's analytic attention, support the emphasis that I am adding here to his conclusions. A comprehensive answer to this question would call for a discussion of the representation of ego interests in dreams. As an example, I can propose only most briefly that in Dora's first dream the *house* and the *jewel case*, besides being symbols of the female body and its contents, represent the adolescent quandary: if there is a fire in "our house" (that is, in our family), then what "valuables" (that is, values) shall be saved first? And indeed, Freud's interpretation, although psychosexual and oedipal in emphasis, assigns to the father standing by the girl's bed not the role of a wished-for seducer but that of a hoped-for protector of his daughter's inviolacy.

Notes

1. W. H. Auden, "Greatness Finding Itself," *Mid-Century* (June 1960), no. 13.

2. Heinz Hartmann, "Notes on the Reality Principle," *The Psychoanalytic Study of the Child* (New York: International Universities Press, 1956), 11:31–53 (italics added).

3. Heinz Loewald, "Ego and Reality," *International Journal of Psychoanalysis* (1951), 32:10–18 (italics added).

4. "There is no simple correlation between the degree of objective insight and the degree of adaptiveness of the corresponding action" (Hartmann, "Notes," p. 40).

5. ["Acting *in regard* to reality" and "action vis-à-vis reality" refer to Hartmann's "Notes" (italics added); "acting *in the outer world*" (italics added) is a phrase from Hartmann, "On Rational and Irrational Action," *Psychoanalysis and the Social Sciences,* (New York: International Universities Press, 1947), 1:359–392.]—Editors' note.

6. The term "actual neurosis" was coined to refer to symptoms caused *directly* by noxious agents of somatic origin. There is also in Freud's papers on metapsychology a mysterious footnote promising a "later passage on the distinction between testing with regard to reality and testing *with regard to immediacy*" ("On the History of the Psycho-analytic Movement," *SE* 14:3–66, italics added). Freud's original terms are *Realitätsprufung* and *Aktualitätsprufung*. To this the editor of the *Standard Edition* adds: "No reference to the latter seems to occur anywhere else; and this may be one more reference to a missing paper." In this address, I will not attempt to surmise what kind of differentiation Freud had in mind; nor can I discuss the formulations of later workers who have concerned themselves with analogous problems without focusing on the points to be made here.

7. Erik H. Erikson, "The First Psychoanalyst," *Yale Review* (1956), 46:40–62. Also in B. Nelson, ed. *Freud and the Twentieth Century* (London: Allen & Unwin, 1957).

8. For a consideration of prolonged adolescence, see P. Blos, "Prolonged Adolescence: The Formation of a Syndrome and Its Therapeutic Implications," *American Journal of Orthopsychiatry* (1954), 24:733–742.

9. Sigmund Freud, "A Metapsychological Supplement to the Theory of Dreams," *SE* 14:217–235. See also D. Rapaport and M. Gill, "The Points of View and Assumptions of Metapsychology," *International Journal of Psychoanalysis* (1959), 40:1–10.

10. Anna Freud, *The Ego and the Mechanisms of Defense* (New York: International Universities Press, 1946).

11. Erik H. Erikson, "Youth: Fidelity and Diversity," *Daedalus* (1962), 91:5–27. See also Erikson, "The Roots of Virtue," in Sir Julian Huxley, ed., *The Humanist Frame* (London: Allen & Unwin, 1961; New York: Harper & Row, 1961).

12. J. Piaget and B. Inhelder, *The Growth of Logical Thinking from Childhood to Adolescence* (New York: Basic Books, 1958).

13. Erik H. Erikson, "The Problem of Ego Identity," *Journal of the American Psychoanalytic Association* (1956), 4:56–121. Also published as *Identity and the Lifecycle*, Monograph, *Psychological Issues*, vol. 1, no. 1 (New York: International Universities Press, 1959).

14. This has been most forthrightly formulated in H. Loewald, "On the Therapeutic Action of Psycho-analysis," *International Journal of Psychoanalysis* (1960), 41:16–33 in which Loewald anticipates much of my argument about the role of reality testing within the actuality of the therapeutic relationship.

3. Freud and Dora: Story, History, Case History

STEVEN MARCUS

It is generally agreed that Freud's case histories are unique. Today more than half a century after they were written they are still widely read. Even more, they are still widely used for instruction and training in psychoanalytic institutes. One of the inferences that such a vigorous condition of survival prompts is that these writings have not yet been superseded. Like other masterpieces of literature or the arts, these works seem to possess certain transhistorical qualities—although it may by no means be easy to specify what those qualities are. The implacable "march of science" has not—or has not yet—consigned them to "mere" history. Their singular and mysterious complexity, density, and richness have thus far prevented such a transformation and demotion.

This state of affairs has received less attention than it merits. Freud's case histories—and his works in general—are unique as pieces or kinds of writing, and it may be useful to examine one of Freud's case histories from the point of view of literary criticism, to analyze it as a piece of writing, and to determine whether this method of proceeding

This essay was first published in *Partisan Review* (Winter 1974). This is a shortened version of the full text, which appears in *Representations* (New York: Random House, 1975), pp. 247–309.

may yield results that other means have not. My assumption—and conclusion—is that Freud is a great writer and that one of his major case histories is a great work of literature. That is to say, it is both an outstanding creative and imaginative performance and an intellectual and cognitive achievement of the highest order. And yet this triumphant greatness is in part connected with the circumstance that it is about a kind of failure, and that part of the failure remains in fact unacknowledged and unconscious.

"Fragment of an Analysis of a Case of Hysteria," better known as the case of Dora, is Freud's first great case history—oddly enough he was to write only four others. It may be helpful for the reader if at the outset I briefly review some of the external facts of the case. In the autumn of 1900, Dora, an eighteen-year-old young woman, began treatment with Freud. She did so reluctantly and against her will, and, Freud writes, "it was only her father's authority which induced her to come to me at all." Neither Dora nor her father were strangers to Freud. He had made separate acquaintance with each of them in the past, during certain episodes of illness that characterized their lives if not the life of the family as a whole. (Freud knew other members of the family as well.)

As for Dora herself, her afflictions, both mental and physical, had begun in early childhood and had persisted and flourished with variations and fluctuating intensities until she was presented to Freud for therapy. Among the symptoms from which she suffered were dyspnea, migraine, and periodic attacks of nervous coughing, often accompanied by complete loss of voice during part of the episode. Dora had in fact first been brought by her father to Freud two years earlier, when she was sixteen and suffering from a cough and hoarseness; he had then "proposed giving her psychological treatment," but this suggestion was not adopted since "the attack in question, like the others, passed off spontaneously." In the course of his treatment of Dora, Freud also learned of further hysterical—or hysterically connected—productions on her part, such as a feverish attack that mimicked appendicitis, a periodic limp, and a vaginal catarrh or discharge. Moreover, during the two-year interval between Dora's first visit and the occasion on which her father brought her to Freud a second time and "handed her over to me for psychotherapeutic treatment . . . Dora had grown unmistakably neurotic." Dora was now "in the first bloom of youth—a girl of intelligent and engaging looks." Her character had, however, undergone an alteration. She had become chronically depressed and was generally dissatisfied with both herself and her family. She had become unfriendly toward the father whom she had hitherto loved, idealized, and identified with. She was "on very bad terms" with her mother, for whom she felt a good deal of scorn. "She tried to avoid social intercourse, and employed herself—so far as she was allowed to by the fatigue and lack of concentration of which she complained—with attending lectures for women and with carrying on more or less serious studies." Two further events precipitated the crisis that led to her being delivered to Freud. Her parents found a written note in which she declared her intention to commit suicide because "as she said, she could no longer endure her life." Following this there occurred one day "a slight passage of words" between Dora and her father that ended with Dora suddenly losing consciousness—the attack, Freud believed, was "accompanied by convulsions and delirious states," although it was lost to amnesia and never came up in the analysis.

Having outlined this array of affections, Freud dryly remarks that such a case "does not upon the whole seem worth recording. It is merely a case of *'petite hystérie'* with the commonest of all somatic and mental symptoms. . . . More interesting cases of hysteria have no doubt been published."

This disavowal of anything sensational to come is of course a bit of shrewd disingenuousness on Freud's part, for what follows at once is his assertion that he is going to elucidate the meaning, origin, and function of every one of these symptoms by means of the events and experiences of Dora's life. He is going, in other words, to discover the "psychological determinants" that will account for Dora's illnesses; among these determinants he lists three principal conditions: "a psychical trauma, a conflict of affects, and . . . a disturbance in the sphere of sexuality." And so Freud begins the treatment by asking Dora to talk about her experiences. What emerges is the substance of the case history, a substance that takes all of Freud's immense analytic, expository, and narrative talents to bring into order. I will again very roughly and briefly summarize some of this material.

Sometime after 1888, when the family had moved to B———, the health resort where the father's tuberculosis had sent them, an intimate and enduring friendship sprang up between them and a couple named K. Dora's father was deeply unhappy in his marriage and apparently made no bones about it. The K.'s too were unhappily married, as it later turned out. Frau K. took to nursing Dora's father during these years of his illness. She also befriended Dora, and they behaved toward one another in the most familiar way and talked together about the most intimate subjects. Herr K., her husband, also made himself a close friend of Dora—going regularly for walks with her and giving her presents. Dora in her turn befriended the K.'s two small children, "and had been almost a mother to them." What begins to be slowly if unmistakably disclosed is that Dora's father and Frau K. had established a sexual liaison and that this relation had by the time of Dora's entering into treatment endured for many years. At the same time Dora's father and Frau K. had tacitly connived at turning Dora over to Herr K., just as years later her father "handed her over to me [Freud] for psychotherapeutic treatment." In some sense everyone was conspiring to conceal what was going on; and in some yet further sense everyone was conspiring to deny that anything was going on at all. What we have here, on one of its sides, is a classical Victorian domestic drama that is at the same time a sexual and emotional can of worms.

Matters were brought to a crisis by two events that happened to Dora at two different periods of her adolescence. When she was fourteen, Herr K. contrived one day to be alone with her in his place of business; in a state of sexual excitement, he "suddenly clasped the girl to him and pressed a kiss on her lips." Dora responded with a "violent feeling of disgust," and hurried away. This experience, like those referred to in the foregoing paragraph, was never discussed with or mentioned to anyone, and relations continued as before. The second scene took place two years later in the summer, when Dora was sixteen (it was just after she had seen Freud for the first time). She and Herr K.

were taking a walk by a lake in the Alps. In Dora's words, as they come filtered to us through Freud, Herr K. "had the audacity to make her a proposal." Apparently he had begun to declare his love for this girl whom he had known so well for so long. "No sooner had she grasped Herr K.'s intention than, without letting him finish what he had to say, she had given him a slap in the face and hurried away." The episode as a whole leads Freud quite plausibly to ask: "If Dora loved Herr K., what was the reason for her refusing him in the scene by the lake? Or at any rate, why did her refusal take such a brutal form, as though she were embittered against him? And how could a girl who was in love feel insulted by a proposal which was made in a manner neither tactless nor offensive?" It may occur to us to wonder whether in the extended context of this case that slap in the face was a "brutal form" of refusal; but as for the other questions posed by Freud, they are without question rhetorical in character.

On this second occasion Dora did not remain silent. Her father was preparing to depart from the Alpine lake, and she declared her determination to leave at once with him. Two weeks later she told the story of the scene by the lake to her mother, who relayed it—as Dora had clearly intended—to her father. In due course Herr K. was "called to account" on this score, but he "denied in the most emphatic terms having on his side made any advances" and suggested that she "had merely fancied the whole scene she had described." Dora's father "believed" the story concocted by Herr—and Frau—K., and it is from this moment, more than two years before she came to Freud for treatment, that the change in Dora's character can be dated. Her love for the K.'s turned into hatred, and she became obsessed with the idea of getting her father to break off relations with them. She saw through the rationalizations and denials of her father and Frau K. and had "no doubt that what bound her father to this young and beautiful woman was a common love-affair. Nothing that could help to confirm this view had escaped her perception, which in this connection was pitilessly sharp." Indeed, "the sharpsighted Dora" was an excellent detective when it came to uncovering her father's clandestine sexual activites, and her withering criticisms of her father's character—that he was "insincere . . . had a strain of baseness in his character . . . only thought of his own enjoyment . . . had a gift for seeing things in the light which suited him best"—were in general concurred in by Freud. Freud also agreed with Dora that there was something in her embittered if exaggerated contention that "she had been handed over to Herr K. as the price of his tolerating the relations between her father and his wife." Nevertheless, the cause of her greatest embitterment seems to have been her father's "readiness to consider the scene by the lake as a product of her imagination." And although Freud was in his customary way skeptical about such impassioned protestations and repudiations—and surmised that something in the way of an opposite series of thoughts or self-reproaches lay behind them—he was forced to come to "the conclusion that Dora's story must correspond to the facts in every respect." If we try to put ourselves in the place of this girl between her sixteenth and eighteenth years, we can at once recognize that her situation was a desperate one. The three adults to whom she was closest, whom she loved the most in the world, were apparently conspiring—separately, in tandem, or in concert—to deny her the reality of her experience. They were conspiring to deny Dora her reality and reality itself. This betrayal touched upon matters that might easily unhinge the mind of a young person; the three adults were not betraying Dora's love and trust alone, they were betraying the structure of the actual world. Indeed, when Dora's father handed her over to Freud with the parting injunction, "Please try and bring her to reason," there were no two ways of taking what he meant. Naturally he had no idea of the mind and character of the physician to whom he had dealt this leading remark.

Dora began treatment with Freud some time in October 1900. Freud wrote to Fliess that "the case has opened smoothly to my collection of picklocks," but the analysis was not proceeding well. The material produced was very rich, but Dora was there more or less against her will. Moreover, she was more than usually amnesic about events in her remote past and about her inner and mental life. The analysis found its focus and climax in two dreams. The first of these was the production by Dora of a dream that in the past she had dreamed recurrently. Among the many messages concealed by it, Freud made out one that he conveyed to his patient: "You have decided to give up the treatment," he told her, adding, "to which, after all, it is only your father who makes you come." It was a self-fulfilling interpretation. A few weeks after the first dream, the second dream occurred. Freud spent two hours elucidating it, and at the beginning of the third, which took place on December 31, 1900, Dora informed him that she was there for the last time. Freud pressed on during this hour and presented Dora with a series of stunning and outrageously intelligent interpretations. The analysis ended as follows: "Dora had listened to me without any of her usual contradictions. She seemed to be moved; she said good-bye to me very warmly, with the heartiest wishes for the New Year, and came no more." Dora's father subsequently called on Freud two or three times to reassure him that Dora was returning, but Freud knew better than to take him at his word. Fifteen months later, in April 1902, Dora returned for a single visit; what she had to tell Freud on that occasion was of some interest, but he knew that she was done with him, as indeed she was.

Dora was actuated by many impulses in breaking off the treatment; prominent among these partial motives was revenge—upon men in general and at that moment Freud in particular, who was standing for those other men in her life who had betrayed and injured her. He writes rather ruefully of Dora's "breaking off so unexpectedly, just when my hopes of a successful termination of the treatment were at their highest, and her thus bringing those hopes to nothing—this was an unmistakable act of vengeance on her part." And although Dora's "purpose of self-injury" was also served by this action, Freud goes on clearly to imply that he felt hurt and wounded by her behavior. Yet it could not have been so unexpected as all that, since as early as the first dream Freud both understood and had communicated this understanding to Dora that she had already decided to give up the treatment. What is suggested by this logical hiatus is that although Dora had done with Freud, Freud had not done with Dora. And this supposition is supported by what immediately followed. As soon as Dora left him, Freud began writing up her case history—a proceeding that, as far as I have been able to ascertain, was not in point of immediacy a usual response for him. He interrupted the composition of the *Psy-*

chopathology of Everyday Life on which he was then engaged and wrote what is substantially the case of Dora during the first three weeks of January 1901. On January 25, he wrote to Fliess that he had finished the work the day before and added, with that terrifying self-confidence of judgment that he frequently revealed, "Anyhow, it is the most subtle thing I have yet written and will produce an even more horrifying effect than usual." The title he had at first given the new work—"Dreams and Hysteria"—suggests the magnitude of ambition that was at play in him. At the same time, however, Freud's settling of his account with Dora took on the proportions of a heroic inner and intellectual enterprise.

Yet that account was still by no means settled, as the obscure subsequent history of this work dramatically demonstrates. In the first letter of January 25, 1901, Freud had written to Fliess that the paper had already been accepted by Ziehen, joint editor of the *Monatsschrift für Psychiatrie und Neurologie*. On the fifteenth of February, in another letter to Fliess, he remarks that he is now finishing up *The Psychopathology of Everyday Life* and that when he has done so he will correct it and the case history. About two months later, in March 1901, according to Ernest Jones, Freud showed "his notes of the case" to his close friend, Oscar Rie. The reception Rie gave to them was such, reports Freud, that "I thereupon determined to make no further effort to break down my state of isolation." On May 8, 1901, Freud wrote to Fliess that he had not yet "made up his mind" to send off the work. One month later, he made up his mind and sent it off, announcing to Fliess that "it will meet the gaze of an astonished public in the autumn." But nothing of the sort was to occur, and what happened next was, according to Jones, "entirely mysterious" and remains so. Freud either sent it off to Ziehen, the editor who had already accepted it, and then having sent it asked for it back. Or he sent it off to another magazine altogether, the *Journal für Psychologie und Neurologie*, whose editor, one Brodmann, refused to publish it. The upshot was that Freud returned the manuscript to a drawer for four more years. And when he did at last send it into print, it was in the journal that had accepted it in the first place.

But we are not out of the darkness and perplexities yet, for when

Freud finally decided in 1905 to publish the case, he revised the work once again. There is one further touch of puzzlements. Freud got the date of his case wrong. When he wrote or rewrote it, either in January 1901 or in 1905, he assigned the case to the autumn of 1899 instead of 1900. And he continued to date it incorrectly, repeating the error in 1914 in the "History of the Psychoanalytic Movement" and again in 1923, when he added a number of new footnotes to the essay on the occasion of its publication in the eighth volume of his *Gesammelte Schriften*. Among the many things suggested by this recurrent error is that in some sense he had still not done with Dora, as indeed I think we shall see he had not. The modern reader may be inclined to remark that these questions of date, of revision, problems of textual status, and authorial uncertainties of attitude would be more suitable to a discussion of a literary text—a poem, play, or novel—than to a work of "science." But such a conception of the nature of scientific discourse—particularly the modes of discourse that are exercised in those disciplines which are not preponderantly or uniformly mathematical or quantitative—has to undergo a radical revision.

The general form of what Freud has written bears certain suggestive resemblances to a modern experimental novel. Its narrative and expository course, for example, is neither linear nor rectilinear; instead its organization is plastic, involuted, and heterogeneous and follows spontaneously an inner logic that seems frequently to be at odds with itself; it often loops back around itself and is multidimensional in its representation of both its material and itself. Its continuous innovations in formal structure seem unavoidably to be dictated by its substance, by the dangerous, audacious, disreputable, and problematical character of the experiences being represented and dealt with, and by the equally scandalous intentions of the author and the outrageous character of the role he has had the presumption to assume. In content, however, what Freud has written is in parts rather like a play by Ibsen, or more precisely like a series of Ibsen's plays. And as one reads through the case of Dora, scenes and characters from such works as *Pillars of Society*, *A Doll's House*, *Ghosts*, *An Enemy of the People*, *The Wild Duck*, and *Rosmersholm* rise up and flit through the mind. There is, however, this difference. In this Ibsen-like drama, Freud is not only Ibsen, the creator and playwright; he is also and directly one of the characters in the action and in the end suffers in a way that is comparable to the suffering of the others.

What I have been reiterating is that the case of Dora is first and last an extraordinary piece of writing, and it is to this circumstance in several of its most striking aspects that we should direct our attention. For it is a case history, a kind or genre of writing—that is to say, a particular way of conceiving and constructing human experience in written language—that in Freud's hands became something that it never was before.

The ambiguities and difficulties begin with the very title of the work, "Fragment of an Analysis of a Case of Hysteria." It is a fragment in the sense that its "results" are "incomplete." The treatment was "broken off at the patient's own wish," at a time when certain problems "had not been attacked and others had only been imperfectly elucidated." It follows that the analysis itself is "only a fragment," as are "the following pages" of writing which present it. To which the modern reader, flushed with the superior powers of his educated irony, is tempted to reply: how is it that this fragment is also a whole, an achieved totality, an integral piece of writing called a case history? And how is it, furthermore, that this "fragment" is fuller, richer, and more complete than the most "complete" case histories of anyone else? But there is no more point in asking such questions of Freud—particularly at this preliminary stage of proceedings—than there would be in posing similar "theoretical" questions to Joyce or Proust.

The work is also fragmentary, Freud continues, warming to his subject, because of the very method he has chosen to pursue; on this plan, that of nondirectional free association, "everything that has to do with the clearing-up of a particular symptom emerges piecemeal, woven into various contexts, and distributed over widely separate periods of time." Freud's technique itself is therefore fragmentary; his way of penetrating to the microstructure—the "finer structure," as he calls it—of a neurosis is to allow the material to emerge piecemeal. At the same time these fragments only *appear* to be incoherent and disparate; in actuality they eventually will be understood as members of a whole.

Furthermore, Freud goes on, there is still another "kind of incompleteness" to be found in this work, and this time it has been "intentionally introduced." He has deliberately chosen not to reproduce "the process of interpretation to which the patient's associations and communications had to be subjected, but only the results of that process." That is to say, what we have before us is not a transcription in print of a tape recording of eleven weeks of analysis but something that is abridged, edited, synthesized, and constructed from the very outset. And as if this were not enough, Freud introduces yet another context in which the work has to be regarded as fragmentary and incomplete. It is obvious, he argues, "that a single case history, even if it were complete and open to no doubt, cannot provide an answer to all questions arising out of the problem of hysteria." Thus, like a modernist writer—which in part he is—Freud begins by elaborately announcing the problematical status of his undertaking and the dubious character of his achievement.

Even more, like some familiar "unreliable narrator" in modernist fiction, Freud pauses at regular intervals to remind the reader of this case history that "my insight into the complex of events composing it [has] remained fragmentary," that his understanding of it remains in some essential sense permanently occluded. This darkness and constraint are the result of a number of converging circumstances, some of which have already been touched on and include the shortness of the analysis and its having been broken off by Dora at a crucial point. But it also includes the circumstances that the analysis—any analysis—must proceed by fragmentary methods, by analyzing thoughts and events bit by discontinuous bit. And at the end of one virtuoso passage in which Freud demonstrates through a series of referential leaps and juxtapositions the occurrence in Dora's past of childhood masturbation, he acknowledges that this is the essence of his procedure. "Part of this material," he writes, "I was able to obtain directly from the analysis, but the rest required supplementing. And, indeed, the method by which the occurrence of masturbation in Dora's case has been verified has shown us that material belonging to a single subject can only be collected piece by piece at various times and in different connections." In sum, the process resembles "reality" itself, a word that, as contemporary writers like to remind us, should always be surrounded by quotation marks.

We are then obliged to ask—and Freud himself more than anyone else has taught us most about this obligation—*what else* are all these protestations of fragmentariness and incompleteness about? They refer in some measure, as Freud himself indicates in the Postscript, to a central inadequacy and determining incompleteness that he discovered only after it was too late—the "great defect" of the case was to be located in the undeveloped, misdeveloped, and equivocal character of the "transference," of the relation between patient and physician in which so much was focused. Something went wrong in the relation between Freud and Dora—or in the relation between Dora and Freud. But the protestations refer, I believe, to something else as well, something of which Freud was not entirely conscious. For the work is also fragmentary or incomplete in the sense of Freud's self-knowledge, both at the time of the actual case and at the time of his writing it. And he communicates in this piece of writing a less than complete understanding of himself, although like any great writer he provides us with the material for understanding some things that have escaped his own understanding, for filling in some gaps, for restoring certain fragments into wholes.

How else can we finally explain the fact that Freud chose to write up this particular history in such extensive detail? The reason that he offers in both the Prefatory Remarks and the Postscript are not entirely convincing—which does not of course deny them a real if fractional validity. Why should he have chosen so problematic a case when presumably others of a more complete yet equally brief kind were available? I think this can be understood in part through Freud's own unsettled and ambiguous role in the case, that he had not yet, so to speak, "gotten rid" of it, that he had to write it out, in some measure, as an effort of self-understanding—an effort, I think we shall see, that remained heroically unfinished, a failure that nonetheless brought lasting credit with it.

If we turn now to the Prefatory Remarks it may be illuminating to regard them as a kind of novelistic framing action, as in these few opening pages Freud rehearses his motives, reasons, and intentions and begins at the same time to work his insidious devices upon the reader. First, exactly like a novelist, he remarks that what he is about to let us in on is positively scandalous, for "the complete elucidation of a case of hysteria is bound to involve the revelation of intimacies and the betrayal of . . . secrets." Second, again like a writer of fiction, he has deliberately chosen persons, places, and circumstances that will remain obscure; the scene is laid not in metropolitan Vienna but "in a remote provincial town." He has from the beginning kept the circumstances that Dora was his patient such a close secret that only one other physician—"in whose discretion I have complete confidence"—knows about it. He has "postponed publication" of this essay for "four whole years," also in the cause of discretion, and in the same cause has "allowed no name to stand which could put a non-medical reader on the scent." Finally he has buried the case even deeper by publishing it "in a purely scientific and technical periodical" in order to secure yet another "guarantee against unauthorized readers." He has, in short, made his own mystery within a mystery, and one of the effects of such obscure preliminary goings-on is to create a kind of Nabokovian frame—what we have here is a history framed by an explanation which is itself slightly out of focus.

Third, he roundly declares, this case history is science and not literature: "I am aware that—in this city, at least—there are many physicians who (revolting though it may seem) choose to read a case history of this kind not as a contribution to the psychopathology of neuroses, but as a *roman à clef* designed for their private delectation." This may indeed be true; but it is equally true that nothing is more literary—and more modern—than the disavowal of all literary intentions. And when Freud does this again later on toward the end of "The Clinical Picture," the situation becomes even less credible. The passage merits quotation at length.

I must now turn to consider a further complication to which I should certainly give no space if I were a man of letters engaged upon the creation of a mental state like this for a short story, instead of being a medical man engaged upon its dissection. The element to which I must now allude can only serve to obscure and efface the outlines of the fine poetic conflict which we have been able to ascribe to Dora. This element would rightly fall a sacrifice to the censorship of a writer, for he, after all, simplifies and abstracts when he appears in the character of a psychologist. But in the world of reality, which I am trying to depict here, a complication of motives, an accumulation and conjunction of mental activities—in a word, overdetermination—is the rule. (*SE* 7:59; *C* 77)

In this context it is next to impossible to tell whether Freud is up to another of his crafty maneuverings with the reader or whether he is actually simply unconscious of how much of a modern and modernist writer he is. For when he takes to describing the difference between himself and some hypothetical man of letters and writer of short stories he is in fact embarked upon an elaborate obfuscation. That hypothetical writer is nothing but a straw man; and when Freud in apparent contrast represents himself and his own activities he is truly representing how a genuine creative writer writes. This passage, we must also recall, came from the same pen that only a little more than a year earlier had written passages about Oedipus and Hamlet that changed for good the ways in which the civilized world would henceforth think about literature and writers.[1] What might be thought of as this sly unliterariness of Freud's turns up in other contexts as well.

If we return to the point in the Prefatory Remarks, we find that Freud then goes on to describe other difficulties, constraints, and problematical circumstances attaching to the situation in which he finds himself. Among them is the problem of "how to record for publication" even such a short case—the long ones are as yet altogether impossible. Moreover, since the material that critically illuminated this case was grouped about two dreams, their analysis formed a secure point of departure for the writing. (Freud is of course at home with dreams, being the unchallenged master in the reading of them.) Yet this tactical solution pushes the *entire problematic* back only another step further, since Freud at once goes on to his additional presupposition, that only those who are already familiar with the interpretation of dreams—that is, *The Interpretation of Dreams* (1900), whose readership in 1901 must have amounted to a little platoon indeed—are likely to be satisfied at all with the present account. Any other reader "will find only bewilderment in these pages." As much as it is like anything else, this is like Borges—as well as Nabokov. This off-putting and disconcerting quality, it should go without saying, is characteristically modern; the writer succumbs to no impulse to make it easy for the reader. On the contrary, he is by preference rather forbidding and does not extend a cordial welcome. The reader has been, as it were, "softened up" by his first encounter with this unique expository and narrative authority; he is thoroughly off balance and is as a consequence ready to be "educated" by Freud. By the same token, however, if he has followed these opening few pages carefully, he is certainly no longer as prepared as he was to assert the primacy and priority of his own critical sense of things. He is precisely where Freud—and any writer—wants him to be.

At the opening of part 1, "The Clinical Picture," Freud tells us that he begins his "treatment, indeed, by asking the patient to give me the whole story of his life and illness," and immediately adds that "the information I receive is never enough to let me see my way about the case." This inadequacy and unsatisfactoriness in the stories his patients tell is in distinct contrast to what Freud has read in the accounts rendered by his psychiatric contemporaries, and he continues by remarking, "I cannot help wondering how it is that the authorities can produce such smooth and exact histories in cases of hysteria. As a matter of fact the patients are incapable of giving such reports about themselves." There is a great deal going on here. In the first place there is the key assumption that everyone—that every life, every existence—has a story, to which there is appended a corollary that most of us probably tell that story poorly. Furthermore, the relations at this point in Freud's prose among the words *story, history,* and *report* are unspecified, undifferentiated, and unanalyzed and in the nature of the case contain and conceal a wealth of material.

Freud proceeds to specify what it is that is wrong with the stories his patients tell him. The difficulties are in the first instance formal shortcomings of *narrative:* the connections, "even the ostensible ones—are for the most part incoherent," obscured and unclear; "and the sequence of different events is uncertain." In short, these narratives are disorganized, and the patients are unable to tell a coherent story of their lives. What is more, he states, "the patients' inability to give an ordered history of their life in so far as it coincides with the history of their illness is not merely characteristic of the neurosis. It also possesses great theoretical significance." What we are led at this juncture to conclude is that Freud is implying that a coherent story is in some manner connected with mental health (at the very least with the absence of hysteria), and this in turn implies assumptions of the broadest and deepest kind about both the nature of coherence and the form and structure of human life. On this reading, human life is, ideally, a connected and coherent story, with all the details in explanatory place, and with everything (or as close to everything as is practically possible) accounted for, in its proper causal or other sequence. Inversely, illness amounts at least in part to suffering from an incoherent story or an inadequate narrative account of oneself.

Freud then describes in technical detail the various types and orders of narrative insufficiency that he commonly finds; they range from disingenuousness, both conscious and unconscious, to amnesias and paramnesias of several kinds and various other means of severing connections and altering chronologies. In addition, he maintains, this discomposed memory applies with particular force and virulence to "the history of the illness" for which the patient has come for treatment. In the course of a successful treatment, this incoherence, incompleteness, and fragmentariness are progressively transmuted as facts, events, and memories are brought into the forefront of the patient's mind. He adds as a conclusion that these two aims "are coincident"—they are reached simultaneously and by the same path. Some of the consequences that can be derived from these extraordinary observations are as follows. The history of any patient's illness is itself only a substory (or a subplot), although it is at the same time a vital part of a larger structure. Furthermore, in the course of psychoanalytic treatment, nothing less than "reality" itself is made, constructed, or reconstructed. A complete story—"intelligible, consistent, and unbroken"—is the theoretical, created end story. It is a story, or a fiction, not only because it has a narrative structure but also because the narrative account has been rendered in language, in conscious speech, and no longer exists in the deformed language of symptoms, the untranslated speech of the body. At the end—at the successful end—one has come into possession of one's own story. It is a final act of self-appropriation, the appropriation by oneself of one's own history. This is in part so because one's own story is in so large a measure a phenomenon of language, as psychoanalysis is in turn a demonstration of the degree to which language can go in the reading of all our experience. What we end with, then, is a fictional construction that is at the same time satisfactory to us in the form of the truth, and as the form of the truth.

No larger tribute has ever been paid to a culture in which the various narrative and fictional forms had exerted for centuries both moral and philosophical authority and that had produced as one of its chief climaxes the great bourgeois novels of the nineteenth century. Indeed, we must see Freud's writings—and method—as themselves part of this culmination, and at the same moment, along with the great modernist novels of the first half of the twentieth century, as the beginning of the end of that tradition and its authority. Certainly the passages we have just dealt with contain heroic notions and offer an extension of heroic capabilities if not to all men then to most, at least as a possibility. Yet we cannot leave this matter so relatively unexamined and must ask ourselves how it is that this "story" is not merely a "history" but a "case history" as well. We must ask ourselves how these associated terms are more intimately related in the nexus that is about to be wound and unwound before us. To begin to understand such questions we have to turn back to a central passage in the Prefatory Remarks. Freud undertakes therein "to describe the way in which I have overcome the *technical* difficulties of drawing up the report of this case history." Apparently the "report" and the "case history" referred to in this statement are two discriminable if not altogether discrete entities. If they are, then we can further presume that, ideally at any rate, Dora (or any patient) is as much in possession of the "case history" as Freud himself. And this notion is in some part supported by what comes next. Freud mentions certain other difficulties, such as the fact that he "cannot make notes during the actual session . . . for fear of shaking the patient's confidence and of disturbing his own view of the material under observation." In the case of Dora, however, this obstacle was partly overcome because so much of the material was grouped about two dreams, and "the wording of these dreams was recorded immediately after the session" so that "they thus afforded a secure point of attachment for the chain of interpretations and recollections which proceeded from there." Freud then writes as follows:

> The case history itself was only committed to writing from memory after the treatment was at an end, but while my recollection of the case was still fresh and was heightened by my interest in its publication. Thus the record is not absolutely—phonographically—exact, but it can claim to possess a high degree of trustworthiness. Nothing of any importance has been altered in it except in some places the order in which the explanations are given; and this has been done for the sake of presenting the case in a more connected form. (*SE* 7:10; *C* 24)

Such a passage raises more questions than it resolves. The first sentence is a kind of conundrum in which case history, writing, and memory dance about in a series of logical entwinements, of possible alternate combinations, equivalences, and semiequivalences. These are followed by further equivocations about "the record," "phonographic" exactitude, and so forth—the ambiguities of which jump out at one as soon as the terms begin to be seriously examined. For example, is "the report" the same thing as "the record," and if "the record" were "phonographically" exact would it be a "report"? Like the prodigious narrative historian that he is, Freud is enmeshed in an irreducible paradox of history: that the term itself refers to both the activity of the historian—the writing of history—and to the objects of his undertaking, what history is "about." I do not think, therefore, that we can conclude that Freud has created this thick context of historical contingency and ambiguity out of what he once referred to as Viennese *schlamperei*.

The historical difficulties are further compounded by several other sequential networks that are mentioned at the outset and that figure discernibly throughout the writing. First there is the virtual Proustian complexity of Freud's interweaving of the various strands of time in the actual account; or, to change the figure, his geological fusing of various time strata—strata that are themselves at the same time fluid and shifting. We observe this most strikingly in the palimpsestlike quality of the writing itself, which refers back to *Studies on Hysteria* of 1895; which records a treatment that took place at the end of 1900 (although it mistakes the date by a year); which then was written up in first form during the early weeks of 1901; which was then exhumed in 1905 and was revised and rewritten to an indeterminable extent before publication in that year; and to which additional critical comments in the form of footnotes were finally appended in 1923. All of these are of course held together in vital connection and interanimation by nothing else than Freud's consciousness.

But we must take notice as well of the copresence of still further different time sequences in Freud's presentation, this copresence being itself a historical or novelistic circumstance of some magnitude. There is first the connection established by the periodically varied rehearsal throughout the account of Freud's own theory and theoretical notions as they had developed up to that point; this practice provides a kind of running applied history of psychoanalytic theory as its development is refracted through the embroiled medium of this particular case. Then there are the different time strata of Dora's own history, which Freud handles with confident and loving exactitude. Indeed, he is never more of a historical virtuoso than when he reveals himself to us as moving with compelling ease back and forth between the complex group of sequential histories and narrative accounts, with divergent sets of diction and at different levels of explanation, that constitute the extraordinary fabric of this work. He does this most conspicuously in his analytic dealings with Dora's dreams, for every dream, he reminds us, sets up a connection between two "factors," an "event during childhood" and an "event of the present day—and it endeavors to reshape the present on the model of the remote past." The existence or recreation of the past in the present is in fact "history" in more than one of its manifold senses and is one of Freud's many analogies to the following equally celebrated utterance.

> Men make their own history, but they do not make it just as they please; they do not make it under circumstances chosen by themselves, but under circumstances directly encountered, given and transmitted from the past. The tradition of all the dead generations weighs like a nightmare on the brain of the living. And just when they seem engaged in revolutionising themselves

and things, in creating something that has never yet existed, precisely in such periods of revolutionary crisis they anxiously conjure up the spirits of the past to their service and borrow from them names, battle cries and costumes in order to present the new scene of world history in this time-honored disguise and this borrowed language. (Marx, *The Eighteenth Brumaire of Louis Bonaparte*)

Just as Marx regards the history makers of the past as sleepwalkers, "who required recollections of past world history in order to drug themselves concerning their own content," so Freud similarly regards the conditions of dream-formation, of neurosis itself, and even of the cure of neurosis, namely, the analytic experience of transference. They are all of them species of living past history in the present. If the last of these works out satisfactorily, then a case history is at the end transfigured. It becomes an inseparable part of an integral life history. Freud is, of course, the master historian of those transfigurations.

At the very beginning, after he had listened to the father's account of "Dora's impossible behavior," Freud abstained from comment, for, he remarks, "I had resolved from the first to suspend my judgement of the true state of affairs till I had heard the other side as well." Such a suspension inevitably recalls an earlier revolutionary project. In describing the originating plan of *Lyrical Ballads,* Coleridge writes that it "was agreed that my endeavours should be directed to persons and characters supernatural, or at least romantic; yet so as to transfer from our inward nature a human interest and a semblance of truth sufficient to procure for these shadows of imagination that willing suspension of disbelief for the moment, which constitutes poetic faith." We know very well that Freud had a more than ordinary capacity in this direction and that one of the most dramatic moments in the prehistory of psychoanalysis had to do precisely with his taking on faith facts that turned out to be fantasies. Yet Freud is not only the reader suspending judgment and disbelief until he has heard the other side of the story; and he is not only the poet or writer who must induce a similar process in himself if he is to elicit it in his audience. He is also concomitantly a principal, an actor, a living character in the drama that he is unfolding in print before us. Moreover, that suspension of disbelief is in no sense incompatible with a large body of assumptions, many of them definite, a number of them positively alarming.

They have to do largely with sexuality and in particular with female sexuality. They are brought to a focus in the central scene of Dora's life (and case), a scene that Freud orchestrates with inimitable richness and to which he recurs thematically at a number of junctures with the tact and sense of form that one associates with a classical composer of music (or with Proust, Mann, or Joyce). Dora told this episode to Freud toward the beginning of their relation, after "the first difficulties of the treatment had been overcome." It is the scene between her and Herr K. that took place when she was fourteen years old—four years before the present tense of the case—and acted Freud said as a "sexual trauma." The reader will recall that on this occasion Herr K. contrived to get Dora alone "at his place of business" in the town of B———, and then without warning or preparation "suddenly clasped the girl to him and pressed a kiss upon her lips." Freud then asserts that "this was *surely* just the situation to call up a *distinct* feeling of sexual excitement in a girl of *fourteen* who had *never before* been approached. But Dora had at that moment a violent feeling of disgust, tore herself free from the man, and hurried past him to the staircase and from there to the street door" (all italics are mine). She avoided seeing the K.'s for a few days after this, but then relations returned to "normal"—if such a term survives with any permissible sense in the present context. She continued to meet Herr K., and neither of them ever mentioned "the little scene." Moreover, Freud adds, "according to her account Dora kept it a secret till her confession during the treatment," and he pretty clearly implies that he believes this.

This episode preceded by two years the scene at the lake that acted as the precipitating agent for the severe stage of Dora's illness; and it was this later episode and the entire structure that she and others had elaborated about it that she had first presented to Freud, who continues thus:

In this scene—second in order of mention, but first in order of time—the behavior of this child of fourteen was already entirely and completely hysterical. I should without question consider a person hysterical in whom an occasion for sexual excitement elicited feelings that were preponderantly or exclusively unpleasurable; and I should do so whether or not the person were capable of producing somatic symptoms. (*SE* 7:28; *C* 44)

Also, in Dora's feeling of disgust an obscure psychical mechanism called the "reversal of affect" was brought into play; but so was another process, and here Freud introduces—casually and almost as a throw-away—one more of his grand theoretical-clinical formulations, namely the idea of the "*displacement* of sensation," or, as it has more commonly come to be referred to, the "displacement upward." "Instead of the genital sensation which would certainly have been felt by a healthy girl in such circumstances, Dora was overcome by the unpleasurable feeling which is proper to the tract of mucous membrane at the entrance to the alimentary canal—that is by disgust." Although the disgust did not persist as a permanent symptom but remained behind residually and potentially in a general distaste for food and poor appetite, a second displacement upward was the resultant of this scene "in the shape of a sensory hallucination which occurred from time to time and even made its appearance while she was telling me her story. She declared that she could still feel upon the upper part of her body the pressure of Herr K.'s embrace." Taking into account certain other of Dora's "inexplicable"—and hitherto unmentioned—"peculiarities" (such as her phobic reluctance to walk past any man she saw engaged in animated conversation with a woman), Freud "formed in my own mind the following reconstruction of the scene. I believe that during the man's passionate embrace she felt not merely his kiss upon her lips but also his erect member against her body. The perception was revolting to her; it was dismissed from her memory, repressed, and replaced by the innocent sensation of pressure upon her thorax, which in turn derived an excessive intensity from its repressed source." This repressed source was located in the erotogenic oral zone, which in Dora's case had undergone a developmental deformation from the period of infancy. And thus, Freud concludes, "the pressure of the erect member probably led to an analogous change in the corresponding female organ, the clitoris; and the excitation of this second erotogenic zone was referred by a process of displacement to the simultaneous pressure against the thorax and became fixed there."

There is something questionable and askew in this passage of unquestionable genius. In it Freud is at once dogmatically certain and very uncertain. He is dogmatically certain of what the normative sexual response in young and other females is, and asserts himself to that effect. At the same time, he is, in my judgment, utterly uncertain about where Dora is, or was, developmentally. At one moment in the passage he calls her a "girl," at another a "child"—but in point of fact he treats her throughout as if this fourteen-, sixteen-, and eighteen-year-old adolescent had the capacities for sexual response of a grown woman. Indeed, at a later point he conjectures again that Dora either responded, or should have responded, to the embrace with specific genital heat and moisture. Too many determinations converge at this locus for us to do much more than single out a few of the more obvious influencing circumstances. In the first instance there was Freud's own state of knowledge about such matters at the time, which was better than anyone else's but still relatively crude and undifferentiated. Second, we may be in the presence of what can only be accounted for by assuming that a genuine historical-cultural change has taken place between then and now. It may be that Freud was expressing a legitimate partial assumption of his time and culture when he ascribes to a fourteen-year-old adolescent—whom he calls a "child"—the normative responses that are ascribed today to a fully developed and mature woman. This supposition is borne out if we consider the matter from the other end, from the standpoint of what has happened to the conception of adolescence in our own time. It begins now in prepuberty and extends to —who knows when? Certainly its extensibility in our time has reached well beyond the age of thirty. Third, Freud is writing in this passage as an advocate of nature, sexuality, openness, and candor—and within such a context Dora cannot hope to look good. The very framing of the context in such a manner is itself slightly accusatory. In this connection we may note that Freud goes out of his way to tell us that he knew Herr K. personally and that "he was still quite young and of prepossessing appearance." If we let Nabokov back into the picture for a moment, we may observe that Dora is no Lolita, and go on to suggest that *Lolita* is an anti-*Dora*.

Yet we must also note that in this episode—the condensed and focusing scene of the entire case history—Freud is as much a novelist as he is an analyst. For the central moment of this central scene is a "reconstruction" that he "formed in [his] own mind." This pivotal construction becomes henceforth the principal "reality" of the case, and we must also observe that this reality remains Freud's more than Dora's, since he was never quite able to convince her of the plausibility of the construction, or, to regard it from the other pole of the dyad, she was never quite able to accept this version of reality, of what "really" happened. Freud was not at first unduly distressed by this resistance on her side, for part of his understanding of what he had undertaken to do in psychoanalysis was to instruct his patients—and his readers—in the nature of reality. This reality was the reality that modern readers of literature have also had to be educated in. It was conceived of as a *world of meanings.* As Freud put it in one of those stop-you-dead-in-your-tracks footnotes that he was so expert in using strategically, we must at almost every moment "be prepared to be met not by one but by several causes—by *overdetermination.*" Thus the world of meanings is a world of multiple and compacted causations; it is a world in which everything has a meaning, which means that everything has more than one meaning. Every symptom is a concrete universal in several senses. It not only embodies a network of significances but also "serves to represent several unconscious mental processes simultaneously." By the same token, since it is a world almost entirely brought into existence, maintained, and mediated through a series of linguistic transactions between patient and physician, it partakes in full measure of the virtually limitless complexity of language, in particular its capacities for producing statements characterized by multiplicity, duplicity, and ambiguity of significance. Freud lays particular stress on the ambiguity, is continually on the lookout for it, and brings his own formidable skills in this direction to bear most strikingly on the analyses of Dora's dreams. The first thing he picks up in the first of her dreams is in fact an ambiguous statement, with which he at once confronts her.

As if this were not sufficient, the actual case itself was full of such literary and novelistic devices or conventions as thematic analogies, double plots, reversals, inversions, variations, and betrayals—full of what the "sharp-sighted" Dora as well as the sharp-sighted Freud thought of as "hidden connections"—although it is important to add that Dora and her physician mean different things by the same phrase. And as the case proceeds Freud continues to confront Dora with such connections and tries to enlist her assistance in their construction. For example, one of the least pleasant characteristics in Dora's nature was her habitual reproachfulness—it was directed mostly toward her father but radiated out in all directions. Freud regarded this behavior in his own characteristic manner: "A string of reproaches against other people," he comments, "leads one to suspect the existence of a string of self-reproaches with the same content." Freud accordingly followed the procedure of turning back "each simple reproach on the speaker herself." When Dora reproached her father with malingering in order to keep himself in the company of Frau K., Freud felt "obliged to point out to the patient that her present ill-health was just as much actuated by motives and was just as tendentious as had been Frau K.'s illness, which she had understood so well." At such moments Dora begins to mirror the other characters in the case, as they in differing degrees all mirror one another as well.

Part of that sense, we have come to understand, is that the writer is or ought to be conscious of the part that he —in whatever guise, voice, or persona he chooses—invariably and unavoidably plays in the world he represents. Oddly enough, although there is none of his writings in which Freud is more vigorously active than he is here, it is precisely this activity that he subjects to the least self-conscious scrutiny, that he almost appears to fend off. For example, I will now take my head in my hands and suggest that his extraordinary analysis of Dora's first dream is inadequate on just this count. He is only dimly and marginally aware of his central place in it (he is clearly incorporated into the figure of Dora's father), comments on it only as an addition to Dora's own addendum to the dream, and does nothing to exploit it. Instead of analyzing his own part in what he has done and what he is writing, Freud continues to behave like an unreliable narrator, treating the material about which he is writing as if it were literature but excluding himself from both that treatment and that material. At one moment he refers to himself as someone "who has learnt to appreciate the delicacy of the fabric of structures such as dreams," intimating what I surmise he incontestably believed, that dreams are natural works of art. And when, in the analysis of the second dream, we find ourselves back at the scene at the lake again, when Dora recalls that the only plea to her of Herr K. that she could remember is "You know I get nothing out of my wife"; when these were precisely the same words used by Dora's father in describing to Freud his relation to Dora's mother; and when Freud speculates that Dora may even "have heard her father make the same complaint . . . just as I myself did from his own lips"—when a conjunction such as this occurs, then we know we are in a novel, probably by Proust. Time has recurred, the repressed has returned, plot, double plot, and counterplot have all intersected, and "reality" turns out to be something that for all practical purposes is indistinguishable from a systematic fictional creation.

Finally, when at the very end Freud turns to deal—rudimentarily as it happens—with the decisive issue of the case, the transferences, everything is transformed into literature, into reading and writing. Transferences, he writes, "are new editions or facsimiles" of tendencies, fantasies, and relations in which "the person of the physician" replaces some earlier person. When the substitution is a simple one, the transferences may be said to be "merely new impressions or reprints": Freud is explicit about the metaphor he is using. Others "more ingeniously constructed . . . will no longer be new impressions, but revised editions." And he goes on, quite carried away by these figures, to institute a comparison between dealing with the transference and other analytic procedures. "It is easy to learn how to interpret dreams," he remarks, "to extract from the patient's associations his unconscious thoughts and memories, and to practise similar explanatory arts: for these the patient himself will always provide the text." The startling group of suppositions contained in this sentence should not distract us from noting the submerged ambiguity in it. The patient does not merely provide the text; he also *is* the text, the writing to be read, the language to be interpreted. With the transference, however, we move to a different degree of difficulty and onto a different level of explanation. It is only after the transference has been resolved, Freud concludes, "that a patient arrives at a sense of conviction of the validity of the connections which have been constructed during the analysis." I will refrain from entering the veritable series of Chinese boxes opened up by that last statement and will content myself with proposing that in this passage as a whole Freud is using literature and writing not only creatively and heuristically—as he so often does—but defensively as well.

The writer or novelist is not the only partial role taken up unconsciously or semiconsciously by Freud in the course of this work. He also figures prominently in the text in his capacity as a nineteenth-century man of science and as a representative Victorian critic—employing the seriousness, energy, and commitment of the Victorian ethos to deliver itself from its own excesses. We have already seen him affirming the positive nature of female sexuality, "the genital sensation which would certainly have been felt by a healthy girl in such circumstances," but which Dora did not feel. He goes a good deal further than this. At a fairly early moment in the analysis he faces Dora with the fact that she has "an aim in view which she hoped to gain by her illness. That aim could be none other than to detach her father from Frau K." Her prayers and arguments had not worked; her suicide letter and fainting fits had done no better. Dora knew quite well how much her father loved her, and, Freud continues to address her:

> I felt quite convinced that she would recover at once if only her father were to tell her that he had sacrificed Frau K. for the sake of her health. But, I added, I hoped he would not let himself be persuaded to do this, for then she would have learned what a powerful weapon she had in her hands, and she would certainly not fail on every future occasion to make use once more of her liability to ill-health. Yet if her father refused to give way to her, I was quite sure she would not let herself be deprived of her illness so easily. (*SE* 7:42; *C* 59)

This is pretty strong stuff, considering both the age and her age. I think, moreover, that we are justified in reading an overdetermination out of this utterance of Freud's and in suggesting that he had motives additional to strictly therapeutic ones in saying what he did.

In a related sense Freud goes out of his way to affirm his entitlement to speak freely and openly about sex—he is, one keeps forgetting, the great liberator and therapist of speech. The passage is worth quoting at some length.

It is possible for a man to talk to girls and women upon sexual matters of every kind without doing them harm and without bringing suspicion upon himself, so long as, in the first place, he adopts a particular way of doing it, and, in the second place, can make them feel convinced that it is unavoidable. . . . The best way of speaking about things is to be dry and direct; and that is at the same time the method furthest removed from the prurience with which the same subjects are handled in "society," and to which girls and women alike are so thoroughly accustomed. I call bodily organs and processes by their technical names. . . . *J'appelle un chat un chat.* I have certainly heard of some people—doctors and laymen—who are scandalized by a therapeutic method in which conversations of this sort occur, and who appear to envy either me or my patients the titillation which, according to their notions, such a method must afford. But I am too well acquainted with the respectability of these gentry to excite myself over them. . . . The right attitude is: "*pour faire une omelette il faut casser des oeufs.*" (*SE* 7:48–9; *C* 65–6)

I believe that Freud would have been the first to be amused by the observation that in this splendid extended declaration about plain speech (at this point he takes his place in a tradition coming directly down from Luther) he feels it necessary to disappear not once but twice into French. I think he would have said that such slips—and the revelation of their meanings—are the smallest price one has to pay for the courage to go on. And he goes on with a vengeance, immediately following this passage with another in which he aggressively refuses to moralize in any condemnatory sense about sexuality. As for the attitude that regards the perverse nature of his patient's fantasies as horrible:

I should like to say emphatically that a medical man has no business to indulge in such passionate condemnation. . . . We are faced by a fact, and it is to be hoped that we shall grow accustomed to it, when we have learned to put our own tastes on one side. We must learn to speak without indignation of what we call the sexual perversions. . . . The uncertainty in regard to the boundaries of what is to be called normal sexual life, when we take different races and different epochs into account, should in itself be enough to cool the zealot's ardor. We surely ought not to forget that the perversion which is the most repellent to us, the sensual love of a man for a man, was not only tolerated by the people so far our superiors in cultivation as were the Greeks, but was actually entrusted by them with important social functions. (*SE* 7:50; *C* 67)

We can put this assertion into one of its appropriate contexts by recalling that the trial and imprisonment of Oscar Wilde had taken place only five years earlier. And the man who is speaking out here has to be regarded as the greatest of Victorian physicians, who in this passage is fearlessly revealing one of the inner and unacknowledged meanings of the famous "tyranny of Greece over Germany." And as we shall see he has by no means reached the limits beyond which he will not go.

How far he is willing to go begins to be visible as we observe him sliding almost imperceptibly from being the nineteenth-century man of science to being the remorseless "teller of truth," the character in a play by Ibsen who is not to be deterred from his "mission." In a historical sense the two roles are not adventitiously related, any more than it is adventitious that the "truth" that is told often has unforeseen and destructive consequences and that it can rebound upon the teller. But we see him most vividly at this implacable work in the two great dream interpretations, which are largely "phonographic" reproductions of dramatic discourse and dialogue. Very early on in the analysis of the first dream, Freud takes up the dream element of the "jewel-case" and makes the unavoidable symbolic interpretation of it. He then proceeds to say the following to this Victorian maiden who has been in treatment with him for all of maybe six weeks.

So you are ready to give Herr K. what his wife withholds from him. That is the thought which has had to be repressed with so much energy, and which has made it necessary for every one of its elements to be turned into its opposite. The dream confirms once more what I had already told you before you dreamt it—that you are summoning up your old love for your father in order to protect yourself against your love for Herr K. But what do all these efforts show? Not only that you are afraid of Herr K., but that you are still more afraid of yourself, and of the temptation you feel to yield to him. In short, these efforts prove once more how deeply you love him. (*SE* 7:70; *C* 88)

He immediately adds that "naturally Dora would not follow me in this part of the interpretation," but this does not deter him for a moment from pressing on with further interpretations of the same order; and this entire transaction is in its character and quality prototypical for the case as a whole. The Freud we have here is not the sage of the Berggasse, not the master who delivered the incomparable *Introductory Lectures* of 1916–1917, not the tragic Solomon of *Civilization and Its Discontents.* This is an earlier Freud, the Freud of the Fliess letters, the Freud of the case of Dora as well. It is Freud the relentless investigator pushing on no matter what. The Freud that we meet with here is a demonic Freud, a Freud who is the servant of his *daimon*. That *daimon* in whose service Freud knows no limits is the spirit of science, the truth, or "reality"—it does not matter which; for him they are all the same. Yet it must be emphasized that the "reality" Freud insists upon is very different from the "reality" that Dora is claiming and clinging to. And it has to be admitted that not only does Freud overlook for the most part this critical difference; he also adopts no measures for dealing with it. The demon of interpretation has taken hold of him, and it is this power that presides over the case of Dora.

In fact, as the case history advances it becomes increasingly clear to the careful reader that Freud and not Dora has become the central character in the action. Freud the narrator does in the writing what Freud the first psychoanalyst appears to have done in actuality. We begin to sense that it is his story that is being written and not hers that is being retold. Instead of letting Dora approprate her own story, Freud became the appropriator of it. The case history belongs progressively less to her than it does to him. It may be that this was an inevitable development, that it is one of the typical outcomes of an analysis that fails, that Dora was under any circumstances unable to become the appropriator of her own history, the teller of her own story. Blame does not necessarily or automatically attach to Freud. Nevertheless, by the time he gets to the second dream he is able to write, "I shall present the material produced during the analysis of this dream in the somewhat haphazard order in which it recurs to my mind." He makes such a presentation for several reasons, most of which are legitimate. But one reason almost certainly is that by this juncture it is his *own* mind that chiefly matters to him, and it is *his* associations to her dream that are of principal importance.

At the same time, as the account progresses, Freud has never been more inspired, more creative, more inventive; as the reader sees Dora gradually slipping further and further away from Freud, the power and complexity of the writing reach dizzying proportions. At times they pass over into something else. Due allowance has always to be made for the absolutizing tendency of genius, especially when as in the case of Dora the genius is writing with the license of a poet and the ambiguity of a seer. But Freud goes beyond this.

When Dora reports her second dream, Freud spends two hours of inspired insight in elucidating some of its meanings. "At the end of the second session," he writes, "I expressed my satisfaction at the results." The satisfaction in question is in large measure self-satisfaction, for Dora responded to Freud's expression of it with the following words uttered in "a depreciatory tone: 'Why, has anything so remarkable come out?' " That satisfaction was to be of short duration, for Dora opened the third session by telling Freud that this was the last time she would be there—it was December 31, 1900. Freud's remarks that "her breaking off so unexpectedly just when my hopes of a successful termination of the treatment were at their highest, and her thus bringing those hopes to nothing—this was an unmistakable act of vengeance on her part" are only partly warranted. There was, or should have been, nothing unexpected about Dora's decision to terminate; indeed, Freud himself on the occasion of the first dream had already detected such a decision on Dora's part and had communicated this finding to her. Moreover, his "highest" hopes for a successful outcome of the treatment seem almost entirely without foundation. In such a context the hopes of success almost unavoidably become a matter of self-reference and point to the immense *intellectual* triumph that Freud was aware he was achieving with the material adduced by his patient. On the matter of "vengeance," however, Freud cannot be faulted; Dora was, among other things, certainly getting her own back on Freud by refusing to allow him to bring her story to an end in the way he saw fit. And he in turn is quite candid about the injury he felt she had caused him. "No one who, like me," he writes, "conjures up the most evil of those half-tamed demons that inhabit the human breast, and seeks to wrestle with them, can expect to come through the struggle unscathed."

This admission of vulnerability, which Freud artfully manages to blend with the suggestion that he is a kind of modern combination of Jacob and Faust, is in keeping with the weirdness and wildness of the case as a whole and with this last hour. That hour recurs to the scene at the lake, two years before, and its aftermath. And Freud ends this final hour with the following final interpretation. He reminds Dora that she was in love with Herr K.; that she wanted him to divorce his wife; that even though she was quite young at the time she wanted "to wait for him, and you took it that he was only waiting till you were grown up enough to be his wife. I imagine that this was a perfectly serious plan for the future in your eyes." But Freud does not say this in order to contradict it or categorize it as a fantasy of the adolescent girl's unconscious imagination. On the contrary, he has very different ideas in view, for he goes on to tell her,

> You have not even got the right to assert that it was out of the question for Herr K. to have had any such intention; you have told me enough about him that points directly towards his having such an intention. Nor does his behavior at L——— contradict this view. After all, you did not let him finish his speech and do not know what he meant to say to you. (*SE* 7:108; *C* 130)

He has not done with her yet, for he then goes on to bring in the other relevant parties and offers her the following conclusion:

> Incidentally, the scheme would by no means have been so impracticable. Your father's relation with Frau K. . . . made it certain that her consent to a divorce could be obtained; and you can get anything you like out of your father. Indeed, if your temptation at L——— had had a different upshot, this would have been *the only possible solution for all the parties concerned.* (*SE* 7:108; *C* 130; italics added)

No one—at least no one in recent years—has accused Freud of being a swinger, but this is without question a swinging solution that is being offered. It is of course possible that he feels free to make such a proposal only because he knows that nothing in the way of action can come of it; but with him you never can tell—as I hope I have already demonstrated. One has only to imagine what in point of ego strength, balance, and self-acceptance would have been required of Dora alone in this arrangement of wife and daughter swapping to recognize at once its extreme irresponsibility, to say the least. At the same time we must bear in mind that such a suggestion is not incongruent with the recently revealed circumstance that Freud analyzed his own daughter. Genius makes up its own rules as it goes along—and breaks them as well. This "only possible solution" was one of the endings that Freud wanted to write to Dora's story; he had others in mind besides, but none of them were to come about. Dora refused or was unable to let him do this; she refused to be a character in the story that Freud was composing for her, and wanted to finish it herself. As we now know, the ending she wrote was a very bad one indeed.

In this extraordinary work Freud and Dora often appear as unconscious, parodic refractions of each other. Both of them insist with implacable will upon the primacy of "reality," although the realities each has in mind differ radically. Both of them use reality, "the truth," as a weapon. Freud does so by forcing interpretations upon Dora before she is ready for them or can accept them. And this aggressive truth bounds back upon the teller, for Dora leaves him. Dora in turn uses her version of reality—it is "outer" reality that she insists upon—aggressively as well. She has used it from the outset against her father, and five months after she left Freud she had the opportunity to use it against the K.'s. In May of 1901 one of the K.'s children dies. Dora took the occasion to pay them a visit of condolence:

> She took her revenge on them. . . . To the wife she said: "I know you have an affair with my father"; and the other did not deny it. From the husband she drew an admission of the scene by the lake which he had disputed, and brought the news of her vindication home to her father. (*SE* 7:121; *C* 143)

She told this to Freud fifteen months after she had departed, when she returned one last time to visit him—to ask him, without sincerity, for further help, and "to finish her story." She finished her story, and as for the rest Freud remarks, "I do not know what kind of help she wanted from me, but I promised to forgive her for having deprived me of the satisfaction of affording her a far more radical cure for her troubles."

But the matter is not hopelessly obscure, as Freud himself has already confessed. What went wrong with the case, "its great defect, which led to its being broken off prematurely," was something that had to do with the transference; and Freud writes, "I did not succeed in mastering the transference in good time." He was, in fact, just beginning to learn about this therapeutic phenomenon, and the present passage is the first really important one about it to have been written. It is also in the nature of things heavily occluded. On Dora's side the transference went wrong in several senses. In the first place there was the failure on her part to establish an adequate positive transference to Freud. She was not free enough to respond to him erotically—in fantasy—or intellectually by accepting his interpretations, both or either of these being prerequisites for the mysterious "talking cure" to begin to work. And in the second, halfway through the case a negative transference began to emerge, quite clearly in the first dream. Freud writes that he "was deaf to this first note of warning," and as a result this negative "transference took me unawares, and, because of the unknown quantity in me which reminded Dora of Herr K., she took her revenge on me as she wanted to take her revenge on him, and deserted me as she believed herself to have been deceived and deserted by him." This is, I believe, the first mention in print of the conception that is known as "acting out"—out of which, one may incidentally observe, considerable fortunes have been made.

We are, however, in a position to say something more than this. For there is a reciprocating process in the analyst known as the countertransference, and in the case of Dora this went wrong too. Although Freud describes Dora at the beginning of the account as being "in the first bloom of youth—a girl of intelligent and engaging looks," almost nothing attractive about her comes forth in the course of the writing. As it unwinds, and it becomes increasingly evident that Dora is not responding adequately to Freud, it also becomes clear that Freud is not responding favorably to this response, and that he does not in fact like Dora very much. He does not like her negative sexuality, her inability to surrender to her own erotic impulses. He does not like "her really remarkable achievements in the direction of intolerable behavior." He does not like her endless reproachfulness. Above all, he does not like her inability to surrender herself to him. For what Freud was as yet unprepared to face was not merely the transference but the countertransference as well—in the case of Dora it was largely a negative countertransference—an unanalyzed part of himself. I should like to suggest that this cluster of unanalyzed impulses and ambivalences was in part responsible for Freud's writing of this great text immediately after Dora left him. It was his way—and one way—of dealing with, mastering, expressing, and neutralizing such material. Yet the neutralization was not complete; or we can put the matter in another way and state that Freud's creative honesty was such that it compelled him to write the case of Dora as he did and that his writing has allowed us to make out in this remarkable fragment a still fuller picture. As I have said before, this fragment of Freud's is more complete and coherent than the fullest case studies of anyone else. Freud's case histories are a new form of literature; they are creative narratives that include their own analysis and interpretation. Nevertheless, like the living works of literature that they are, the material they contain is always richer than the original analysis and interpretation that accompany it, and this means that future generations will recur to these works and will find in them a language they are seeking and a story they need to be told.

Note

1. Some years earlier Freud had been more candid and more innocent about the relation of his writing to literature. In *Studies on Hysteria* he introduces his discussion of the case of Fräulein Elisabeth von R. with the following disarming admission:

"I have not always been a psychotherapist. Like other neuropathologists, I was trained to employ local diagnoses and electro-prognosis, and it still strikes me myself as strange that the case histories I write should read like short stories and that, as one might say, they lack the serious stamp of science. I must console myself with the reflection that the nature of the subject is evidently responsible for this, rather than any preference of my own. The fact is that local diagnosis and electrical reactions lead nowhere in the study of hysteria, whereas a detailed description of mental processes such as we are accustomed to find in the works of imaginative writers enables me, with the use of a few psychological formulas, to obtain at least some kind of insight into the course of that affection." (*SE* 2:160)

4. Intervention on Transference

JACQUES LACAN

The objective of the present article is once again to accustom people's ears to the term *subject*. The individual providing us with this opportunity will remain anonymous, which will avoid my having to document all the passages clearly distinguishing him in what follows.

Had one wished to consider the question of Freud's part in Dora's case as closed, then there might be an overall advantage to be gained from this attempt to reopen the study of transference, on the appearance of the report presented under that title by Daniel Lagache.[1] His originality was to account for it by "the Zeigarnik effect," an idea bound to please at a time when psychoanalysis seemed short of alibis.[2]

When the colleague, who shall be nameless, took the credit of replying to the author of the report that one could equally well claim the presence of transference within this effect, I took this as an opportune moment to speak of psychoanalysis.

This essay was presented as a paper to the Congress of Romance-Language Psychoanalysts in 1951. It was first published in the *Revue française de psychanalyse* (1952), and then in Lacan's *Ecrits* (Paris: Seuil, 1966), pp. 215–226. The present translation was made by Jacqueline Rose for inclusion in *Feminine Sexuality: Jacques Lacan and the Ecole Freudienne*, Juliet Mitchell and Jacqueline Rose, eds. (New York: Norton, 1983). The opening section is Lacan's own introduction to the reprinting of the essay in *Ecrits*.

I have had to go back on this, since I was moreover way in advance here of what I have stated since on the subject of transference.

By commenting that the Zeigarnik effect would seem to depend more on transference than to be determinant of it, our colleague B introduced what could be called the "facts of resistance" into psychotechnic experiment. Their import is the full weight they give to the primacy of the relationship of subject to subject in all reactions of the individual, inasmuch as these are human, and to the predominance of this relationship in any test of individual dispositions, whether the conditions of that test are defined as a task or as a situation.

What needs to be understood regarding psychoanalytic experience is that it proceeds entirely in a relationship of subject to subject—which means that it preserves a dimension irreducible to all psychology considered as the objectification of certain properties of the individual.

What happens in an analysis is that the subject is, strictly speaking, constituted through a discourse, to which the mere presence of the psychoanalyst brings, before any intervention, the dimension of dialogue.

Whatever irresponsibility, or even incoherence, the ruling conventions might impose on the principle of this discourse, it is clear that these are merely strategies of navigation (*D* 15; *P* 45; *C* 30–31) intended to ensure the crossing of certain barriers, and that this discourse must proceed according to the laws of a gravitation peculiar to it, which is called truth.[3] For "truth" is the name of that ideal movement which discourse introduces into reality. Briefly, *psychoanalysis is a dialectical experience,* and this notion should predominate when one poses the question of the nature of transference.

In this sense my sole objective will be to show, by means of an example, the kind of proposition to which this line of argument might lead. I will, however, first allow myself a few remarks that strike me as urgent for the present guidance of our work of theoretical elaboration, remarks that concern the responsibilities conferred on us by the moment of history we are living, no less than by the tradition entrusted to our keeping.

The fact that a dialectical conception of psychoanalysis has to be presented as an orientation peculiar to my thinking must surely indicate a failure to recognize an immediate given, that is, the self-evident fact that it deals solely with *words*, while the privileged attention paid to the function of the mute aspects of behavior in the psychological maneuver merely demonstrates a preference on the part of the analyst for a point of view from which the subject is no more than an object. If, indeed, there be such a misrecognition, then we must question it according to the methods we would apply in any similar case.

It is known that I am given to thinking that at the moment when the perspective of psychology, together with that of all the human sciences, was thrown into total upheaval by the conceptions originating from psychoanalysis (even if this was without their consent or even their knowledge), then an inverse movement appeared to take place among analysts, which I would express in the following terms.

Whereas Freud took it upon himself to show us that there are illnesses which speak (unlike Hesiod, for whom the illnesses sent by Zeus descended on mankind in silence), and to convey the truth of what they are saying, it seems that, as the relationship of this truth to a moment in history and a crisis of institutions becomes clearer, the greater the fear it inspires in the practitioners who perpetuate its technique.

Thus, in any number of forms, ranging from pious sentiment to ideals of the crudest efficiency, through the whole gamut of naturalist propaedeutics, they can be seen sheltering under the wing of a psychologism that, in its reification of the human being, could lead to errors besides which those of the physician's scientism would be mere trifles.

For precisely on account of the strength of the forces opened up by analysis, nothing less than a new type of alienation of man is coming into being, as much through the efforts of collective belief as through the selective process of techniques with all the formative weight belonging to rituals: in short, a *homo psychologicus*—a danger I would warn you against.

It is in relation to him that I ask you whether we will allow ourselves to be fascinated by his fabrication or whether, by rethinking the work of Freud, we cannot retrieve the authentic meaning of his initiative and the way to maintain its beneficial value.

Let me stress here, should there be any need, that these questions are in no sense directed at the work of someone like our friend Lagache: the prudence of his method, his scrupulous procedure, and the openness of his conclusions are all exemplary of the distance between our *praxis* and psychology. I will base my demonstration on the case of Dora because of what it stands for in the experience of transference when this experience was still new, this being the first case in which Freud recognized that the analyst played his part [see note 3].

It is remarkable that up to now nobody has commented that the case of Dora is set out by Freud in the form of a series of dialectical reversals. This is not a mere contrivance for presenting material whose emergence Freud clearly states here is left to the will of the patient. What is involved is a scansion of structures in which truth is transmuted for the subject, affecting not only her comprehension of things but her very position as subject of which her "objects" are a function. This means that the conception of the case history is *identical* to the progress of the subject, that is, to the reality of the treatment.

Now, this is the first time Freud gives the term *transference* as the concept for the obstacle on which the analysis broke down. This alone gives at the very least the value of a return to sources to the examination I will be conducting of the dialectical relations that constituted the moment of failure. Through my examination, I will be attempting *to define in terms of pure dialectics the transference,* which we call negative on the part of the subject, as being the operation of the analyst who interprets it.

We will, however, have to go through all the phases that led up to this moment, while also tracing through them all the problematic insights that, in the given facts of the case, indicate at what points it might have had a successful outcome. Thus we find:

A first development, exemplary in that it carries us straight onto the plane where truth asserts itself. Thus, having tested Freud out to see if he will show himself to be as hypocritical as the paternal figure, Dora enters into her indictment, opening up a dossier of memories whose rigor contrasts to the lack of biographical precision characteristic of neurosis. Frau K. and her father have been lovers for years, concealing the fact with what are at times ridiculous fictions. But what crowns it all is that Dora is thus left defenseless against the attentions of Herr K., to which her father turns a blind eye, thus making her the object of an odious exchange.

Freud is too wise to the consistency of the social lie to have been duped by it, even from the mouth of a man he considers owing him a total confidence. He therefore had no difficulty in removing from the mind of the patient any imputation of complicity over this lie. But at the end of this development he is faced with the question, which is moreover classical in the first stage of a treatment: "This is all perfectly correct and true, isn't it? What do you want to change in it?" To which Freud's reply is:

A first dialectical reversal, wanting nothing of the Hegelian analysis of the protest of the "beautiful soul," which rises up against the world in the name of the law of the heart: "Look at your own involvement," he tells her, "in the disorder which you bemoan" (*D* 36; *P* 67; *C* 51). What then appears is:

A second development of truth: namely, that it is not only on the basis of her silence, but through the complicity of Dora herself and, what is more, even under her vigilant protection, that the fiction had been able to continue that allowed the relationship of the two lovers to carry on. What can be seen here is not simply Dora's participation in the courtship of which she is the object on the part of Herr K. New light is thrown on her relationship to the other partners of the quadrille by the fact that it is caught up in a subtle circulation of precious gifts, serving to compensate the deficiency in sexual services, a circulation that starts with her father in relation to Frau K., and then comes back to the patient through the liberality it releases in Herr K. Not that this stands in the way of the lavish generosity that comes to her directly from the first source, by way of parallel gifts, this being the classic form of honorable redress through which the bourgeois male has managed to combine the reparation due to the legitimate wife with concern for the patrimony (note that the presence of the wife is reduced here to this lateral appendage to the circuit of exchange).

At the same time it is revealed that Dora's oedipal relation is grounded in an identification with her father, which is favored by the latter's sexual impotence and is, moreover, felt by Dora as a reflection on the weight of his position as a man of fortune. This is betrayed by the unconscious allusion that Dora is allowed by the semantics of the word *fortune,* in German: *Vermögen.* As it happens, this identification showed through all the symptoms of conversion presented by Dora, a large number of which were removed by this discovery.

The question then becomes: in the light of this, what is the meaning of the jealousy that Dora suddenly shows toward her father's love affair? The fact that this jealousy presents itself in such a *supervalent* form, calls for an explanation that goes beyond its apparent motives (*D* 54–55; *P* 88–89; *C* 71–72). Here takes place:

The second dialectical reversal, which Freud brings about by commenting that, far from the alleged object of jealousy providing its true motive, it conceals an interest in the person of the subject-rival, an interest whose nature, being much less easily assimilated to common discourse, can only be expressed within it in this inverted form. This gives rise to——

A third development of truth: the fascinated attachment of Dora for Frau K. ("her adorable white body" [*D* 61; *P* 96; *C* 79]), the extent to which Dora was confided in, up to a point that will remain unfathomed, on the state of her relations with her husband, the blatant fact of their exchange of friendly services, which they undertook like the joint ambassadoresses of their desires in relation to Dora's father.

Freud spotted the question to which this new development was leading.

If, therefore, it is the loss of this woman that you feel so bitterly, how come you do not resent her for the additional betrayal that it was she who gave rise to those imputations of intrigue and perversity in which they are all now united in accusing you of lying? What is the motive for this loyalty that makes you hold back the last secret of your relationship? (that is, the sexual initiation, readily discernible behind the very accusations of Frau K.). This secret brings us to:

The third dialectical reversal: the one that would yield to us the real value of the object that Frau K. is for Dora. That is, not an individual, but a mystery, a mystery of her femininity, by which I mean her bodily femininity—as it appears uncovered in the second of the two dreams whose study makes up the second part of Dora's case history, dreams to which I suggest you refer in order to see how far their interpretation is simplified by my commentary.

The boundary post that we must go around to complete the final reversal of our course already appears within reach. It is that most distant of images that Dora retrieves from her early childhood (note that the keys always fall into Freud's hands even in those cases which are broken off, like this one). The image is that of Dora, probably still an *infans*, sucking her left thumb, while with her right hand she tugs at the ear of her brother, her elder by a year and a half (*D* 51 and 21; *P* 85 and 51; *C* 69 and 35).

What we seem to have here is the imaginary matrix in which all the situations developed by Dora during her life have since come to be cast—a perfect illustration of the theory of repetition compulsion, whch was yet to appear in Freud's work. It gives us the measure of what woman and man signify for her now.

Woman is the object which it is impossible to detach from a primitive oral desire, and yet in which she must learn to recognize her own genital nature. (One wonders here why Freud fails to see that the aphonia brought on during the absences of Herr K. [*D* 39–40; *P* 71–72; *C* 55–56] is an expression of the violent appeal of the oral erotic drive when Dora was left face to face with Frau K., without there being any need for Freud to invoke her awareness of the fellatio undergone by the father [*D* 47–48; *P* 80–81; *C* 64–65] when everyone knows that cunnilingus is the artifice most commonly adopted by "men of means" whose powers begin to abandon them.) For Dora to gain access to this recognition of her femininity, she would have to take on this assumption of her own body, failing which she remains open to the functional fragmentation (to refer to the theoretical contribution of the mirror stage) that constitutes conversion symptoms.

Now, if she were to fulfill the condition for this access, the original *imago* shows us that her only opening to the object was through the intermediary of the masculine partner, with whom, because of the slight difference in years, she was able to identify, in that primordial identification through which the subject recognizes itself as I. . . .

So Dora had identified with Herr K., just as she is in the process of identifying with Freud himself. (The fact that it was on waking from her dream "of transference" that Dora noticed the smell of smoke belonging to the two men does not indicate, as Freud said [*D* 73; *P* 109; *C* 91–92], a more deeply repressed identification, but much more that this hallucination corresponded to the dawning of her reversion to the *ego.)* And all her dealings with the two men manifest that aggressivity which is the dimension characteristic of narcissistic alienation.

Thus it is the case, as Freud thinks, that the return to a passionate outburst against the father represents a regression as regards the relationship started up with Herr K.

But this homage, whose beneficial value for Dora is sensed by Freud, could be received by her as a manifestation of desire only if she herself could accept herself as an object of desire, that is to say, only once she had worked out the meaning of what she was searching for in Frau K.

As is true for all women, and for reasons that are at the very basis of the most elementary forms of social exchange (the very reasons that Dora gives as the ground for her revolt), the problem of her condition is fundamentally that of accepting herself as an object of desire for the man, and this is for Dora the mystery motivating her idolatry for Frau K. Just so in her long meditation before the Madonna, and in her recourse to the role of distant worshiper, Dora is driven toward the solution Christianity has given to this subjective impasse, by making woman the object of a divine desire, or else, a transcendent object of desire, which amounts to the same thing.

If, therefore, in a third dialectical reversal, Freud had directed Dora toward a recognition of what Frau K. was for her, by getting her to confess the last secrets of their relationship, then what would have been his prestige (this merely touches on the meaning of positive transference)—thereby opening up the path to a recognition of the virile object? This is not my opinion, but that of Freud (*D* 120; *P* 120; *C* 141–142).

But the fact that his failure to do so was fatal to the treatment is attributed by Freud to the action of the transference (*D* 116–20; *P* 157–62; *C* 137–42), to his error in putting off its interpretation (*D* 118;

P 160; *C* 140), when, as he was able to ascertain after the fact, he had only two hours before him in which to avoid its effects (*D* 119; *P* 161; *C* 141).

But each time he comes back to invoking this explanation (one whose subsequent development in analytic doctrine is well known), a note at the foot of the page goes and adds an appeal to his insufficient appreciation of the homosexual tie binding Dora to Frau K.

What this must mean is that the second reason strikes him as the most crucial only in 1923, whereas the first bore fruit in his thinking from 1905, the date when Dora's case study was published.

As for us, which side should we come down on? Surely that of crediting him on both counts by attempting to grasp what can be deduced from their synthesis.

What we then find is this. Freud admits that for a long time he was unable to face this homosexual tendency (which he nonetheless tells us is so constant in hysterics that its subjective role cannot be overestimated) without falling into a perplexity (*D* 120 *n.* 1; *P* 162 *n.* 1; *C* 142 *n.* 1) that made him incapable of dealing with it satisfactorily.

We would say that this has to be ascribed to prejudice, exactly the same prejudice that falsifies the conception of the Oedipus complex from the start, by making it define as natural, rather than normative, the predominance of the paternal figure. This is the same prejudice we hear expressed simply in the well-known refrain, "As thread to needle, so girl to boy."

Freud feels a sympathy for Herr K. that goes back a long way, since it was Herr K. who brought Dora's father to Freud (*D* 19; *P* 49; *C* 33–34) and this comes out in numerous appreciative remarks (*D* 29 *n.* 3; *P* 60 *n.* 3; *C* 44 *n.* 15). After the breakdown of the treatment, Freud persists in dreaming of a "triumph of love" (*D* 109–10; *P* 151–52; *C* 131–32).

As regards Dora, Freud admits his personal involvement in the interest she inspires in him at many points in the account. The truth of the matter is that it sets the whole case on edge, breaking through the theoretical digression, and elevating this text, among the psychopathological monographs that make up a genre of our literature, to the tone of a Princesse de Clèves trapped by a deadly blocking of utterance.[4]

It is because he put himself rather too much in the place of Herr K. that, this time, Freud did not succeed in moving the Acheron.

Because of his countertransference, Freud keeps reverting to the love that Herr K. might have inspired in Dora, and it is odd to see how he always interprets as confessions what are in fact the very varied responses that Dora argues against him. The session when he thinks he has reduced her to "no longer contradicting him" (*D* 104; *P* 145; *C* 125) and that he feels able to end by expressing to her his satisfaction, Dora in fact concludes on a very different note. "Why, has anything so very remarkable come out?" she says, and it is at the start of the following session that she takes her leave of him.

What, therefore, happened during the scene of the declaration at the lakeside, the catastrophe upon which Dora entered her illness, leading everyone to recognize her as ill—this, ironically, being their response to her refusal to carry on as the prop for their common infirmity (not all the "gains" of a neurosis work solely to the advantage of the neurotic)?

As in any valid interpretation, we need only stick to the text to understand it. Herr K. could get in only a few words, decisive though they were: "My wife is nothing to me." The reward for his effort was instantaneous: a hard slap (whose burning aftereffects Dora felt long after the treatment in the form of a transitory neuralgia) gave back to the blunderer: "If she is nothing to you, then what are you to me?"

And after that what will he be for her, this puppet who has nonetheless just broken the enchantment under which she had been living for years?

The latent pregnancy fantasy which follows on from this scene cannot be argued against our interpretation, since it is a well-known fact that it occurs in hysterics precisely as a function of their virile identification.

It is through the very same trap door that Freud will disappear, in a sliding which is even more insidious. Dora withdraws with the smile of the Mona Lisa, and even when she reappears, Freud is not so naive as to believe her intention is to return.

At this moment she has got everyone to recognize the truth, which, while it may be truthful, she knows does not constitute the final truth, and she then manages through the mere *mana* of her presence to precipitate the unfortunate Herr K. under the wheels of a carriage. The abatement of her symptoms, brought about during the second phase of the treatment, did however last. Thus the arrest of the dialectical process is sealed by an obvious retreat, but the positions reverted to can only be sustained by an assertion of the *ego,* which can be taken as an improvement.

Finally, what is this transference whose work Freud states somewhere goes on invisibly behind the progress of the treatment, and whose effects, furthermore, are "not susceptible to definite proof?" (*D* 74; *P* 110; *C* 92). Surely in this case it can be seen as an entity altogether relative to the countertransference, defined as the sum total of the prejudices, passions, and difficulties of the analyst, or even of his insufficient information, at any given moment of the dialectical process. Does not Freud himself tell us (*D* 118; *P* 160; *C* 140) that Dora might have transferred onto him the paternal figure had he been fool enough to believe in the version of things the father had presented to him?

In other words, the transference is nothing real in the subject other than the appearance, in a moment of stagnation, of the analytic dialectic, of the permanent modes according to which it constitutes its objects.

What, therefore, is meant by interpreting the transference? Nothing other than a ruse to fill in the emptiness of this deadlock. But while it may be deceptive, this ruse serves a purpose by setting off the whole process again.

Thus, even though Dora would have denied any suggestion of Freud's that she was imputing to him the same intentions as had been displayed by Herr K., this denial would have done nothing to change the scope of its effects. The very opposition to which it would have given rise would probably, despite Freud, have set Dora off in the favorable direction: that which would have led her to the object of her real interest.

And the fact of setting himself up personally as a substitute for Herr K. would have saved Freud from overinsisting on the value of the marriage proposals of the father.

Thus transference does not arise from any mysterious property of affectivity, and even when it reveals an emotive aspect, this only has meaning as a function of the dialectical moment in which it occurs.

But this moment is of no great significance since it normally translates an error on the part of the analyst, if only that of wishing too much for the good of the patient, a danger Freud warned against on many occasions.

Thus analytic neutrality takes its true meaning from the position of the pure dialectician who, knowing that all that is real is rational (and vice versa), knows that all that exists, including the evil against which he struggles, corresponds as it always will to the level of his own particularity and that there is no progress for the subject other than through the integration that he arrives at from his position in the universal: technically through the projection of his past into a discourse in the process of becoming.

The case of Dora is especially relevant for this demonstration in that, since it involves a hysteric, the screen of the *ego* is fairly transparent—there being nowhere else, as Freud has said, where the threshold is lower between the unconscious and the conscious, or rather, between the analytic discourse and the *word* of the symptom.

I believe, however, that transference always has this same meaning of indicating the moments where the analyst goes astray, and equally takes his or her bearings, this same value of calling us back to the order of our role—that of a positive nonacting with a view to the orthodramatization of the subjectivity of the patient.

Notes

1. Daniel Lagache, "Some Aspects of Transference," *International Journal of Psycho-analysis* (1953), 34(1):1–10—Translator's note.

2. Briefly, this consists of the psychological effect produced by an unfinished task when it leaves a Gestalt in suspense: for instance, that of the generally felt need to give to a musical bar its rhyming chord.

3. Lacan announces at a subsequent point in his text, where we have inserted "[see note 3]," "So that the reader can check my commentary in its textual detail, wherever I refer to Freud's case study, reference is given in the text to the translation published by Denoël and to the 1954 P.U.F. edition in a footnote." Although we have been unable to consult the Denoël edition, in the cases where Lacan's reference is clearly identifiable the pagination of that translation corresponds closely, and is indeed usually identical, to that of the *Standard Edition*. Our references to the

Collier edition are based on this correspondence. We refer first to the Denoël edition (abbreviated *D*), then to the *Pelican Freud*, vol. 8, with the page number furnished by Jacqueline Rose in her translation, and finally to the Collier edition—Editors' note.

4. Madame de Lafayette, *La Princesse de Clèves* (Paris: Claude Barbin, 1678). This novel has always had in France the status of a classic. What is relevant here is that it is taken up almost entirely with the account of a love that is socially and morally unacceptable; and at the decisive moment in the plot, the heroine confesses to her husband, who, previously a model of moral generosity, is destroyed by the revelation—Translator's note.

5. The Scene of Psychoanalysis
The Unanswered Questions of Dora

SUZANNE GEARHART

In the debate that continues to surround Freud's work, he is seen by some as the founder of an authentic science and by others as a thinker who attempted to give scientific status to a set of inherited social and political values. The psychoanalytic phenomenon of transference has provided a focal point in this debate between Freud's critics, and in particular between his feminist critics and certain of his partisans. For the former, Freud never wholly succeeds in overcoming his limitations as an individual—his historical and social limitations and, ultimately, even his own desires. The result, for these critics, is that he never adequately analyzes the problem of countertransference, that is, the distortion or bias imposed on his psychoanalytic theory and practice by those limitations and desires. For Jacques Lacan, on the other hand, the countertransference is the negative phase of a dialectical process that leads, practically speaking, to the positive transference—the key to all successful analyses—and, theoretically speaking, to an ultimately coherent, unified, scientific theory. This debate is a highly significant one, for it relates not only to all phases of psychoanalytic interpretation

This essay was first published in *Diacritics* (Spring 1979), pp. 114–126 where it appeared as a review essay dealing with Lacan's "Intervention sur le transfert" and Luce Irigaray's *Speculum de l'autre femme* (Paris: Minuit, 1974).

but, moreover, to all theories of society insofar as they imply a theory of sexual difference. More significant than what divides Freud's critics and his defenders, however, is what unites them. Even the critical interpreters of Freud have accepted the argument of Freud's partisans, in particular the assumptions at the basis of transference, by continuing to privilege the principle of paternity according to which Freud is the author, the master, the sovereign subject, and ultimately the father of his work. Among Freud's case histories, *Dora* has solicited the attention of interpreters who have seen the issue of transference as vital to the larger question of the scientific claims Freud made for his work, for although Dora's treatment was to fail, according to Freud due to his inability to recognize and to deal with the transference, the case nonetheless represents the beginning of Freud's effort to determine the theoretical status of transference. For our purposes, the Dora case represents neither the immanence of Freud, the scientist, who would in the last instance be responsible for the unity of his work, nor of a Freud who would be the passive medium of an autonomous sociohistorical process, but, rather, an interrogation of the principle of paternity—the symbolic status of the father—both as the key to the "ultimate" explanation of Dora's illness and as the basis of the identity of Freud and his work.

In a much-cited letter to Fliess, Freud described a turning point in his theory of the role of the father in the etiology of hysteria. "Let me tell you straight away the great secret that has been slowly dawning on me in recent months. I no longer believe in my neurotica. . . . There was the definite realization that there is no 'indication of reality' in the unconscious, so that it is impossible to distinguish between truth and emotionally charged fiction."[1] Freud and Breuer's original hypothesis had been that hysteria stemmed from a memory so distressing to consciousness that it had of necessity to be repressed, thus becoming both unconscious and pathogenic. Freud had also found, however, that in the case of the hysteric this memory was, more often than not, not just any memory but the memory of a seduction of the patient by her father. But as the number of cases cured or not cured by the cathexis of this particular memory increased, Freud's belief in the reality of his patients' accusations diminished. Whereas Freud's early theory of hysteria had been based on the reality of the seduction scene, by the time of his letter to Fliess he had come to regard the seduction scene as a fantasy or screen that was itself in need of interpretation. The historical reality of the child's relation to her father was no longer the central question. The imaginary—if not symbolic—nature of that relationship was clear. Freud thus came to see the scene of seduction as a knife that cut both ways. The accusation against the father went with and concealed an accusation directed by the patient against herself—that she had desired a child by her own father.

The "return to Freud" inaugurated by Jacques Lacan has served to underscore the fundamental importance of Freud's remarks to Fliess. This is especially clear in Lacan's interpretation of the Dora case in "Intervention sur le transfert" (see essay 4), for the psychoanalytic procedure of treating even coherent, logical accusations on the patient's part as screens or symptoms was first set down there.[2] The role of this procedure in Freud's analysis of Dora and its implications for psychoanalysis as a whole provide the focal point for Lacan's interpretation of the Dora case.

According to Lacan's analysis, Freud's interpretation of Dora's illness begins with the turning back of her accusations against her, a procedure that Lacan calls the "reversal of the *beautiful soul*" (the term comes from Hegel's *Phenomenology;* just how this borrowing indebts Lacan to Hegel will be discussed further on). But in asking what benefits Dora derives from a situation she describes as objective, as existing independently of her will or interests, Freud cannot fail to find his own interpretation of Dora's illness put to a similar test. The theoretical validity of Freud's procedure hinges on the result of this test, and Lacan takes care to show that, in certain respects, Freud must be said to have failed. Under ideal circumstances, Freud would have remained aloof from the scene by the lake between Herr K. and Dora, which is at the center of his analysis of Dora. In fact, as even Freud himself admits, he became implicated in the scene through a countertransference onto Herr K., and the theoretical consequences of this countertransference are evident, for Lacan, in the relative single-mindedness with which Freud repeatedly brings his interpretation of Dora's illness back to her relationship with Herr K.

Lacan's point, however, is that while Freud's personal and historical limitations may have blinded him to the psychoanalytic consequences of this countertransference, the neutral perspective from which the problems it caused could have been resolved is still discoverable in Freud's exposition of the case: "In Freud's observations, even those which like this one, are cut short, don't all the keys always fall into his hands?"[3] Lacan's defense of Freud's handling of the Dora case invokes a distinction between a Freud who still in some sense believes that the scene that is the focus of his analysis has a historical referent and a Freud who nonetheless succeeds in uncovering the imaginary, nonreferential nature of that scene. For Lacan, the ultimate effect of the countertransference is not to implicate Freud in the Dora case but rather to open the way to a transcendence of his historical role in it. In this sense, the countertransference exists only to permit the emergence of a (positive) transference.

> What is this transference after all? . . . Cannot it be considered to be an entity entirely relative to the countertransference defined as the sum of the prejudices, the passions, the difficulties . . . of the analyst at a given moment of the dialectical process? . . . What does it mean, then, to interpret the transference? Nothing other than to fill this dead space with a decoy. But this decoy is useful, for though it misleads, it restarts the process. (p. 225; *p. 102*)

In the sense that Lacan's analysis of Dora hinges on a distinction between an actor implicated in the scene and a neutral position not directly implicated in it, "Intervention sur le transfert" restates the principal themes of the "return to Freud," and *Dora* and the seduction scene around which Freud's interpretation of the case is organized come to represent and to repeat the "primal scene" of psychoanalysis—the scene that in a sense condenses the whole of the Oedipus phase and in which the castration of the little girl is revealed to the children of both sexes.[4] Up until the event of this scene, the little boy believes that there is only one (masculine) sex and that each of its members possesses a penis. The scene itself, then, can have two effects, one imaginary, one symbolic. Insofar as the scene merely reassures the little boy that, although the little girl may be "castrated," he himself still possesses his sex, insofar as he continues to believe that the measure of sexuality—the phallus—and the penis are one and the same, the effect of the scene is said to be imaginary.[5] Insofar as the scene reveals to the little boy that his own sex is contingent, that the phallus and the penis are not the same, the scene becomes the "pivot" of a symbolic process: "Freud unveiled this imaginary function of the phallus as the pivot of a symbolic process which is brought to its completion *for both sexes* by the putting into question of (the) sex by the castration complex" (p. 555). It is because his work unveils the imaginary nature of the phallus that Freud, for Lacan, must be distinguished from the little boy who persists in his denial of castration through a variety of psychic mechanisms (fetishism, forclusion, etc.). Freud's countertransference onto Herr K. implicates him in the scene of psychoanalysis, but he still holds all the keys. For Lacan, the distinction between the Imaginary and the Symbolic, between the subject who is caught up in the imaginary relationships described by the scene and the (position of the) analyst, is absolute, even if the knowledge of the "little boy"/actor is in some sense retained by the analyst. The phallus, like the seduction scene in whose historical reality Freud has ceased to believe, is a value without a referent, natural or ideal, except from the mystified perspective of the little boy or of the Freud of the countertransference.

In Lacan's analysis of the Dora case, the distinction between the Symbolic and the Imaginary,[6] between the Freud of the countertransference and the Freud of the transference, functions implicitly as a refutation of a feminist critique of psychoanalysis. Feminists have found Dora a particularly sympathetic figure, and this is not surprising when one considers that Freud's strategy with Dora—that of turning her rational indictment of her father back against her—was precisely that adopted by Freud toward the feminists' indictment of a masculine bias of psychoanalysis:

> It is to be anticipated that men analysts with feminist views, as well as . . . women analysts, will disagree with what I have said here. They will hardly fail to object that such notions spring from the "masculinity complex" of the male and are designed to justify on theoretical grounds his innate inclination to disparage and suppress women. But this sort of psychoanalytic argumen-

tation reminds us here, as it does so often, of Dostoevsky's famous "knife that cuts both ways." The opponents of those who argue in this way will on their side think it quite natural that the female sex would refuse to accept a view which appears to contradict their eagerly coveted equality with men. The use of analysis as a weapon of controversy can clearly lead to no decision. ("On Female Sexuality," *SE* 21: 230)

The use of the distinction between the Symbolic and the Imaginary as a defense of psychoanalysis against feminist accusations becomes explicit in Moustapha Safouan's *La sexualité féminine dans la doctrine freudienne* (Paris: Seuil, 1976), which contains a direct response to Luce Irigaray's analysis of the "masculine bias" of psychoanalysis in her *Speculum de l'autre femme*. Safouan turns to the Lacanian distinction between the Symbolic and the Imaginary in order, if not to refute, then to limit the pertinence of Irigaray's analysis of the castration scene. Safouan says of the scene in question:

That this absence should signify "castration" to him [the little boy] can only result from an interpretation. . . . If it is thus, it is because the kid already desires the little girl he observes. . . . [The experience of castration] is indeed a new one, but it is not a perceptual experience: rather it is the experience of desire. (Safouan, p. 80)

Safouan attempts to refute Irigaray's argument by assenting to it in part. Insofar as the castration of the little girl is perceived from the imaginary perspective of the little boy, it would indeed be subject to Irigaray's critique. But the fact that, for Safouan, the castration scene represents the experience of *desire* means that it belongs to a different, Symbolic order, and this fact neutralizes castration, making it impossible to criticize or to analyze it as a value.

Although Safouan's argument may have merit with respect to some feminist writing on psychoanalysis, its application to Irigaray raises some questions. Indeed, Irigaray distinguishes her own position from that characteristic of Freud's feminist critics, for, as Irigaray sees it, their critique of Freud is aimed at demonstrating that women are equally capable of representing phallic values since those values are culturally and not biologically defined. In this sense, their attack has been aimed only at the Freud of the countertransference, whose pronouncements are not always consistent with the insights of his letter to Fliess and who at times assigns to the phallus a natural referent that his theory as a whole, according to Lacan, shows is absent. In contrast to these critics, the focus of Irigaray's analysis is the value that feminists, in disputing Freud, have continued to respect. The scene that opens (and closes) the phallic phase in the child of either sex occupies a central position in Irigaray's critique of Freud, not simply because it fixes the sexual destiny of each child (the adult's sexual and social comportment being traceable to the role played in it) but because it naturalizes a whole system of phallic values by grafting them on to a "perception" that is already part and parcel of that system. In denouncing the complicity of this perception of sexual difference and this set of values, Irigaray does not pretend, at least immediately, to speak in the name of "another" perception or "other" values. For Irigaray, the scene in question is not merely the representation of certain values that happen to be phallic, it is the representation of the conditions of the existence of any value whatsoever.

The perception of castration that serves as the content of the scene is not just one thing among others that can be perceived by the subject. This perception is the condition of the existence of the subject, and as such it determines the subject as essentially masculine: "All theories of the 'subject' will always have been appropriated by the 'masculine.' . . . The subjectivity denied to the woman is, without doubt, the condition which guarantees the constitution of any object: object of representation, of discourse, of desire" (Irigaray, p. 165). The scene of castration has only one subject then, as the concept of "penisneid" implies. The little girl will have seen herself through the eyes of the little boy; she, like the little boy, will have no knowledge of nor attach any value to her "invisible" or "less visible" sex. It is on this ground that Irigaray challenges the absolute nature of the distinction between the little boy and the (position of) the analyst. For though the little boy may confound penis and phallus, he knows one thing the analyst knows—he knows the truth of the little girl's sex, the truth-as-castration. This fundamental identity is the basis of the oppositions articulated by the scene—between the Imaginary and the Symbolic, between the Freud of the countertransference (or the little boy) and the Freud who holds all the keys, the Freud of the transference.

Irigaray's critical analysis of psychoanalysis confirms in its way the decisiveness of the turning point described by Freud in his letter to Fliess, in which the structural as opposed to the historical significance of the seduction scene becomes evident. Decisive as this point is for Freud, it is doubtless even more so for Lacan in that it serves as the authority for his claim to be rescuing Freud from the general effects of the countertransference on his work, while at the same time remaining faithful, more faithful than Freud himself, to Freud's own doctrine. In the case of Dora, the status of two fundamental concepts of psychoanalysis—transference and bisexuality—is "blurred" by what Lacan will analyze as the effects of the countertransference. My aim is to follow the process by which Lacan's discussion of these two concepts rescues the Freud of the transference from the Freud of the countertransference, to analyze the conditions under which this process takes place, and to raise the questions that Lacan's recuperation of the countertransference leaves unanswered.

For Lacan, the principal psychoanalytic concept of which the Dora case is an exposé is that of transference—his references to the case invariably mention it in this light. The enigma of the case, in his view, is in the relationship between the theme of transference and the theme of homosexuality, which is stated only at the very end of the case. Each problem is at various times named by Freud as the factor that led to Dora's analysis being broken off prematurely, and yet, as Lacan points out, no attempt is made by Freud to synthesize the two themes. In Lacan's view, the key to Freud's failure to do so lay in "his prejudice which from the beginning falsifies the conception of the Oedipus complex by making him [Freud] consider as natural, rather than normative, the prevalence of the paternal figure" (p. 223; *p. 100*). Although in other respects Freud's handling of Dora's case is consistent with the revelations of his letter to Fliess, in certain respects, according to Lacan, Freud remained a prisoner of the notion that the "paternal figure" did have a natural referent. According to this erroneous view, the repressed attraction of Dora for Herr K., which Freud initially viewed as the mainspring of her illness, would be a reflection of her Oedipal love for her father, and this love itself would ultimately reflect the "natural" attraction of the opposite sexes for each other and the father's "natural" position as the first member of the opposite sex known to the infant girl. In the light of such an interpretation, Dora's homosexuality could appear only as a disruptive, incoherent element.

The concept that was to resolve Freud's perplexity in the face of female homosexuality was that of identification. By the time of the *Three Introductory Lectures* (1905), Freud had ceased to view the choice of a sexual partner as a natural, objective phenomenon. Freud's analysis of homosexuality had convinced him both of the "nonobjective" nature of the object choice and of the existence of an underlying bisexual disposition in men and women that could account for deviations from the "norm" of heterosexuality. This bisexual disposition was in turn based on the capacity of the subject to identify with either partner in an imagined sexual scene:

> The assumption of a bisexual predisposition in man is particularly clearly brought out by psychoanalysis of neurotics. A quite analogous situation occurs when anyone in his conscious masturbatory phantasies pictures himself both as the man and as the woman in an imagined situation; further counterparts of this are found in certain hysterial attacks in which the patient acts at one and the same time both parts of the underlying sexual phantasy. ("Hysterical Phantasies and Their Relation to Bisexuality," *SE* 9:165–66; *C* 151).

Lacan sees this principle of identification at work in the scene by the lake, in which Dora is both participant and spectator. Because she is both, she identifies equally with Herr K. and with his feminine partner, who is Frau K. by law but who, in this instance, is Dora herself. This identification establishes a certain equivalence between masculinity and femininity. Her own sexual identity and that of Herr K. both become roles, devoid of any natural referent that would prevent Dora from assuming or oblige her to assume that identity. It is in the light of this dual identification that Lacan interprets the scene by the lake.[7] For him, Herr K.'s declaration, "I get nothing from my wife," is interpreted by Dora as indicating a lack in his wife. But what

Dora's identification with Herr K. permits her to see is that this lack is not specific to Frau K. or more generally to women. This is a fundamental lack—a (symbolic) castration—that affects both the masculine and feminine roles. While Herr K.'s declaration expresses only contempt for his wife, according to Lacan, Dora immediately recognizes that his contempt, by right, should extend to Herr K. himself.

Interpreted in this way, the scene by the lake makes clear Freud's "mistake" in his dealings with Dora. For if the purpose of his analysis was to bring Dora to a "recognition of the virile object," the scene by the lake reveals that Herr K. was not a sufficient instrument of such a recognition. "*Fantoche,*" a marionette, a shadow of the virile object (or its "natural referent"), is what, in Lacan's interpretation, Herr K. rightly becomes for Dora. The result of the scene by the lake is revealed to be identical to the result of the scene in which the castration of the little girl is revealed for both sexes. Each is the "pivot of a symbolic process which is brought to its completion *for both sexes* by the putting into question of (the) sex by the castration complex" (p. 555). Thus while Freud's countertransference blinds him to the relationship between Dora's homosexuality and the symbolic process that is the basis of transference, Dora's rejection of Herr K.'s proposal demonstrates a superior, if not ultimate, insight into the relationship between the two themes. While Freud envisages a "practical" solution of Dora's nervous problems—marriage to Herr K., etc.—Dora's simultaneous identification with the masculine and feminine roles in the scene by the lake makes clear the imaginary nature of the "virile object" and, thereby, of Freud's identification with Herr K. Ultimately Freud could have been identified with Frau K. as well as Herr K.; Dora's homosexual love itself could have been transferred to Freud. The transference and the problem posed by Dora's homosexuality could (only) have been mastered simultaneously:

> Thus, if, in a third dialectical reversal, Freud had oriented Dora towards the recognition of what Mme K. was for her . . . by obtaining a confession of the ultimate secrets of her [Dora's] relationship to her [Frau K.], his own prestige would have benefited greatly (we are at this point only beginning to pose the question of the sense of the positive transference), thus opening the way to the recognition of the virile object. (p. 222; *p.* 99)

For Lacan, Herr K.'s desire for Dora and the "interest" of the analyst for her are only shadows of the desire of which "she" is ultimately the object. And if Dora desires an object, that object is neither Herr K. nor Frau K. but the transcendent object that her identification with each entails:

> The problem of her [feminine] condition is at bottom to accept herself as an object of man's desire, and this is, for Dora, the mystery which motivates her idolatry of Mme. K., . . . just as, in her long meditation in front of the painting of the Madonna . . . it [the problem of her condition] pushes her towards the solution which Christianity has given to the subjective impasse, by making the woman the object of a divine desire or, what amounts to the same thing, a transcendent object of desire. (p. 222; *p.* 99)

This is the conclusion toward which the Dora case tends, according to Lacan, even though Freud, due to his countertransference, is unable to come to it himself. The countertransference veils the truth of the Dora case, but this function itself is necessary in the ultimate unveiling of the truth—"for though it misleads, it restarts the process."

But the countertransference, like the text it determines, can only play this role if it is carefully watched, only if it is carefully confined within a dialectic that preordains its sense and limits its potentially disruptive effects, only if the unity and originality of the scene of sexual difference are maintained. Lacan's interpretation of the relationship between the countertransference and (positive) transference, between the theme of bisexuality and of transference, and between the text of the Dora case and the truth of psychoanalysis leaves several aspects of the Dora case unexplained. Lacan's analysis does not take into consideration all the inconsistencies of Dora, and it must be asked if those he neglects can be analyzed within the framework elaborated in "Intervention sur le transfert."

Luce Irigaray has focused on many of these "inconsistencies," and for her they are symptomatic of a certain disarray that characterizes Freud's pronouncements on the issue of feminine sexuality. She traces these inconsistencies to various sources. The imminence of Freud's own death and "a 'scientific honesty' on Freud's part which exists beyond all doubt" (Irigaray, pp. 74–75) may have provoked remarks that call into question the fundamental tenets of his theory of feminine sexuality, and his own unconscious may have been responsible for a failure of his writings on the subject of feminine sexuality to live up to the logical prescriptions he set for himself as a scientist. Indeed, on certain points—notably with respect to his "deconstruction" of the concept of presence—Irigaray sees Freud as the eminent critic of the system of representation underlying his own theory of sexuality. In formulating his theory of sexual difference he is nonetheless, for Irigaray, "prisoner himself of a certain economy of language, of a certain logic, notably where 'desire' is concerned, whose link to classical philosophy he 'misunderstands,' . . . caught up in an 'ideology' which he does not question" (Irigaray, pp. 28–29). Thus any inconsistencies in Freud's work are for Irigaray subordinate to the figure of a Freud who controls his work and who, in this sense, can be accused of not having "put *sufficiently* into question . . . an economy of representation to which he has recourse" (Irigaray, p. 55, italics added). Irigaray's analysis of the question of feminine sexuality forcefully demonstrates the strategic value of the critique of the subject, and yet, in one important form she respects the notion: for Irigaray, the name "Freud" designates a totality in whose name the "contradictions" of the work can be reduced. Although in important respects her critique opposes her to Lacan, in this sense Irigaray participates in a "return to Freud." The Freud who guarantees the coherence of the Dora case for Lacan is the same Freud called to account by Irigaray. While there may be strategic reasons for respecting in Freud's case a concept whose authority she questions everywhere else, Irigaray never discusses them, and the status of "Freud" in this sense falls outside the scope of her critique of the subject. One may ask, therefore, if the inconsistencies that exist in *Dora* can be reduced in the name of a subject that, as the tool of a critical strategy, itself escapes scrutiny, any more than in the name of the subject of a positive transference.

To begin with, one must ask if the case of *Dora* relates the themes of female homosexuality and of transference in the way Lacan says: "But each time he again invokes this explanation [that he failed to recognize and to master the transference in good time], . . . a note appears at the bottom of the page which duplicates it by referring to his insufficient appreciation of the homosexual link between Dora and Mme. K." (p. 223; *p. 100*). In Lacan's view, the text of *Dora*—the procedures adopted by Freud in combining the theoretical and narrative aspects of the case as well as the problems unresolved by this procedure—is determined by the countertransference, that is, by the historical and personal limitations of Freud. Thus for Lacan the fact that Freud's remarks on homosexuality appear only as footnotes to the passages on transference is explainable by the development of Freud's thought between 1905, "date of publication of the Dora case," and 1923, the date of the addition of the footnotes. Freud's failure to synthesize the two themes in *Dora* itself would thus be anecdotal and devoid of any theoretical consequences.

And yet if the importance of a bisexual disposition of the libido fundamental to both normal sexuality and to the various forms of neurosis was evident to Freud at a later date, one would expect later analyses dealing with these problems to have a different result. Indeed, by the time of the *Three Introductory Lectures* (1905), Freud writes, the presence of a homosexual current in the unconscious life of hysterics and neurotics was a firmly established hypothesis.[8] And yet, judging from the "Psychogenesis of a Case of Homosexuality in a Woman" (1920), Freud continued to view female homosexuality as a psychic current that, although it did not exclude the development of the transference, at least under certain circumstances did exclude any possibility of the transference acquiring a positive sense:

> It seemed, further, as though nothing resembling a transference to the physician had been effected. That, however, is of course absurd, or, at least, is a loose way of expressing it; for some kind of relation to the analyst must come about, and this is usually transferred from an infantile one. In reality she transferred to me the deep antipathy to men which had dominated her ever since the disappointment she had suffered from her father. . . . So as soon as I recognized the girl's attitude to her father, I broke off the treatment and gave the advice that, if it was thought worthwhile to continue the therapeutic efforts, it should be done by a woman. (*SE* 18:164)

The resistance that female homosexuality opposes in this case to the development of a positive transference causes Freud to fall back on the "natural prejudice" ("natural" in the sense of "common," and in the sense that this prejudice views the father as a natural rather than normative figure) that was the source of his failings with Dora. Freud's feeling that the young lesbian's attitude toward him has a natural determinant (apparent in his advice that, if her analysis has any chance of success, it would only be with a woman analyst) recalls his hope that Dora's hysteria would find a natural solution—in marriage to Herr K. or to some other young man. Twenty years after his failure to synthesize the themes of transference and female homosexuality (bisexuality) in his analysis of Dora, Freud once again presents himself as incapable of integrating the current of female homosexuality into the dynamic transference that would transcend its strictly negative phase.

That female homosexuality is still experienced by Freud as an absolute obstacle in the "Psychogenesis of a Case of Homosexuality in a Woman" casts doubt on Lacan's assertion that a positive transference could have begun to emerge in the case of *Dora* from the moment Freud had obtained "the confession of the ultimate secrets" of Dora's relation to Frau K. Lacan views the hypothesis of an analysis "based on the principle that all of its formulations are systems of defense" as an aberration that would result in, or be the sign of, a total disorientation of the patient (leaving us free to speculate as to what such a situation would mean for the analyst) and affirms that Freud's interpretation of Dora's illness "does not present these dangers" (p. 305). And yet the theme of female homosexuality as exposed in these two case studies does seem to endanger the theoretical preeminence of the positive transference, which, in Lacan's interpretation, bestows upon the Dora case the coherence it lacked under Freud's pen.

Within *Dora* itself, the theme of bisexuality, which is in question in Freud's discussion of female homosexuality, is not entirely exhausted by Lacan's interpretation—that it points the way toward the development of a positive transference. Freud treats the problem of bisexuality explicitly only in his discussion of Dora's homosexual relation to Frau K. Lacan takes over this circumscription of the problem by carrying out his own analysis of *Dora* within the framework of three "dialectical reversals." This dialectical framework, as well as the critique of the *beautiful soul,* which, for Lacan, opens Freud's analysis of

Dora, constitute a significant borrowing from Hegel's *Phenomenology*, and like all "exchanges" between Lacanian psychoanalysis and the history of philosophy, this one takes place only accompanied by the most careful precautions. Lacan's reinterpretation of the relationship between psychoanalysis and the history of philosophy exhibits a distinction which parallels that between the Freud of the countertransference and the Freud of the transference, between the Imaginary and the Symbolic. There is a history of philosophy of which psychoanalysis is a part. "You have heard me . . . refer with respect and admiration to Descartes and to Hegel. It is fashionable nowadays to 'go beyond' the classical philosophers. . . . Neither Socrates, nor Descartes, nor Marx, nor Freud can be 'gone beyond' in that they have conducted their research with that passion to uncover which has an object: the truth" (p. 193). Psychoanalysis carries on a philosophical tradition extending from Plato to Heidegger and retains its "truth." But where that tradition was fascinated and even deluded by idealism, psychoanalysis permits the unveiling of what that idealism tended to mask: a "dead space," a "lack," the truth-as-castration.

Lacan's comment on the *Aufhebung* of Hegelian dialectics typifies the distinction that for him exists between psychoanalysis and the history of philosophy and reveals the qualifications to which his use of Hegel in "Intervention sur le transfert" is subject: "It is our own *Aufhebung* which transforms that of Hegel, his being a decoy [by which, Lacan hints, he himself was fooled] into an opportunity to *relever* [that is, both to point out and to *aufheben*, or to synthesize in the Hegelian sense] instead of and in the place of the leaps forward of an ideal progress, the ups and downs [or transformations] of a lack" (p. 837). In Lacan's view, Hegel's own critique of idealism in the section of *Phenomenology* dealing with Kant, Fichte, and the German romantics does not prevent the *Phenomenology* itself from being implicated in that idealism in the form of the *Aufhebung*.

Even if one accepts Lacan's distinction between the ideal or the *Aufhebung* on the one hand and the Symbolic order that organizes the unconscious on the other, the consequences of Lacan's borrowings from the *Phenomenology* cannot be entirely neutralized. The Hegelian dialectic provides Lacan with the methodological authority that facilitates one of the most critical aspects of his interpretation: his schematization of the relationship between Dora's heterosexual desires and her homosexual ones. The analysis that is designed to show the synthetic relationship between the two unconscious currents begins by pigeonholing each current in a discrete stage of the dialectical process. The result is that the second (homosexual) current can appear only as derived from the first.

The issue of bisexuality is restricted to the second dialectical stage and can only be raised once the first dialectical stage is "complete," that is, only once Dora's logical, rational account of her situation has been scrutinized in every detail from the standpoint of the psychic benefits Dora herself derives from it. But one aspect of Dora's version of her family history is never scrutinized, although it is duly noted by Freud. This notation implicitly raises the issue of bisexuality from the beginning of the case, and in a manner that disrupts the dialectical schema of Lacan. "Dora," writes Freud, "looked down on her mother and used to criticize her mercilessly, and she had withdrawn completely from her influence" (*SE* 7:20; *C* 35). Dora's opinion of her mother and her interpretation of their relationship differ insignificantly from Freud's own view, but unlike the rest of her story, the "truth," of this assertion will not be scrutinized for its value as an alibi. And this, despite the fact that the case was written up when the concurrence of female homosexuality in the etiology of Dora's hysteria was clear:

> I never made her mother's acquaintance. From the account given me by the girl and her father I was led to imagine her as an uncultivated woman and above all a foolish one, who had concentrated all her interests upon domestic affairs. . . . She had no understanding of her children's more active interests, and was occupied all day long in cleaning the house and its furniture and in keeping them clean—to such an extent as to make it almost impossible to use or enjoy them. (*SE* 7:20; *C* 34).

Freud's treatment of Dora's relationship to her mother is faithful to the account of the infant girl's development he was to present thirty years later in "Female Sexuality." In both places, the girl's "preoedipal" phase is conceived in terms of her ulterior relationship to the phallic values that, with the onset of the Oedipus complex, will attach themselves to what Lacan calls the "paternal metaphor." But what is particularly interesting about the evocation of the patient's relationship to her mother in *Dora* is the fact that Freud's view of that relationship and Dora's view of it mirror each other. The "reversal of the *beautiful soul,*" the total putting into question of Dora's version of things, is thus not as systematic as one is led to believe. Prior to the countertransference onto Herr K., which is to provide Freud with all his insights but which will cause the analysis to end prematurely, is at least a partial countertransference onto Dora herself, through the identity of aspects of Freud's and Dora's representations of her illness. The "secret" of this identity is as carefully guarded by Freud as the secret of her attachment to Frau K. is by Dora: "Her father, then, had fallen ill through leading a loose life, and she assumed that he had handed on his bad health to her by heredity. I was careful not to tell her that, as I have already mentioned, I was of the opinion too, that the offspring of luetics were very specially predisposed to severe neuro-psychoses" (*SE* 7:75; *C* 93). Indeed, if Dora's relationship to Freud demonstrates "that aggressivity in which we can discern the proper dimension of narcissistic alienation" (p. 222; *p. 99*), what of Freud's relation to Dora? Her last act is to give Freud fifteen days' notice—to treat him like a maidservant. The details of her story fully document Freud's interpretation of this point. Freud's own last act is to (re)name Dora, for considerations of social propriety prevented Freud from publishing the case under his patient's actual name. The name he chose was—tit for tat—that of the Freuds' maid, who, like Dora, had been "obliged" to renounce her own name (*The Psychopathology of Everyday Life, SE* 6:241–42).

The uneven execution of the "reversal of the *beautiful soul*" puts into question both the "integrity" of Freud's countertransference onto Herr K. and the triadic structure that provides the framework for Lacan's dialectical analysis of the case. The "prejudice" concerning the natural referent of the Oedipus complex, which had to be disposed of in order to come to terms with the homosexual current of hysteria, finds refuge in the restriction of the problem of countertransference to Freud's relationship to Herr K. It is with the analysis of the phenomenon of countertransference that the prejudice concerning the natural referent of the Oedipus complex is itself naturalized. The prejudice, in a process characteristic of denial, is broken down into two parts. It is considered no longer credible (negation), but its very negation permits the retention of the belief itself, as a "prejudice," and in this form it becomes the basis of the coherence and unity of the dialectical process, which, for Lacan, gives form to *Dora*. The countertransference, however, cannot be restricted to Freud's identification with Herr K. It manifests itself in an identification with Dora as well and thus disrupts the unity of the dialectical process it was intended, in its simple form, to guarantee.

There is (at least) one other direction in which the countertransference exceeds the limits assigned to it by Lacan and by Freud himself. Lacan writes that the transference is an entity "entirely relative to the countertransference defined as the sum of the prejudices, the passions, the difficulties, and even the insufficient information of the analyst at a given moment of the dialectical process" (p. 225; *p. 102*). According to this formula, Dora's attitude toward Freud is the complement of his countertransference. But Freud gives several indications that the transference of "the paternal figure" onto Freud is more prevalent in the Dora case than Lacan suggests. If the transference and countertransference are indeed complementary, as Lacan affirms, one is forced to conclude that Freud's countertransference was not restricted to Herr K. but that there was a countertransference onto Dora's father as well and that, despite Lacan's affirmations, the former does not necessarily exclude the latter. Lacan writes: "Does not Freud himself tell us that Dora could have transferred onto him the paternal figure, if he had been stupid enough to believe the version of things with which Dora's father had presented him?" (p. 225; *p. 102*). "Thus he had no trouble putting out of his patient's mind any imputation of complacency as regards this lie [that is, Dora's father's version of things]" (p. 219; *p. 96*). But Freud himself writes that "at the beginning it was clear that I was replacing her father in her imagination" (*SE* 7:118; *C* 140). It is only with the narration of the second dream that Freud can decisively state that he has come to occupy the place of Herr K. in Dora's imagination, that is, six weeks into an analysis that was to last only twelve weeks. As for the exclusive character that Lacan ascribes to the countertransference, it is clear that Dora's transference of her attitude toward Herr K. onto Freud is not incompatible with the transference of her attitude toward her father onto Freud. Freud and Herr K. are often coupled by both Freud himself and by Lacan without it being evident why Dora's father (as well as Dora herself) should not be included in the series. The perception of an odor of smoke will be traced back to Freud and to Herr K. But Dora's father is a smoker (as is Dora herself). Dora's relations to Freud and Herr K. are characterized by "that aggressivity in which we can discern the proper dimension of narcissistic alienation" (p. 222; *p.* 99). But not more than her relationship to her own father is characterized by such aggressivity. Her homosexual love for Frau K. certainly reinforces her identification with Herr K., but how could it not equally reinforce an identification with her father, whose relation to Frau K. was as intimate as that of the husband?

The justification for putting aside the father in this series will be that Dora's "love" for him is reactive, that is, it is a part of her neurotic defense against Herr K.'s attentions (p. 222; *p.* 99). But Freud argues this point from a position that his statements on bisexuality reveal after the fact to be only partially valid:

> For years on end she had given no expression to this passion for her father. On the contrary, she had for a long time been on the closest terms with the woman who had supplanted her with her father, and she had actually . . . facilitated this woman's relations with her father. Her own love for her father had therefore been recently revived . . . clearly as a reactive symptom, so as to suppress something else. (*SE* 7:57–8; *C* 75)

Freud's own statements on the hysteric's identification with both actors in an imagined sexual scene indicate that Dora's cooperation in Frau K.'s affair with her father would not necessarily imply a waning of her oedipal attitude toward him and that it could even be a means of fostering that attitude. Her relationship to the couple certainly has a homosexual component. But that relationship could also serve as a means of reappropriating and securing the place Frau K. had usurped from her, through an identification with Frau K.

The insistence with which Lacan's interpretation of the countertransference pushes Herr K. to the fore must be compared to his insistence in pushing Dora's father into the background—and ultimately off the stage. Indeed, one can say that it is the distinction between the two figures that maintains the distinction between the inside of the scene of psychoanalysis and its outside—thus making that scene visible to the theorizing glance of the psychoanalyst. For Dora's father to enter onto the stage as an actor would be to run the risk of a fundamental blurring of the distinction between himself and Herr K. and, thereby, of a fundamental disruption of the unity and coherence of the scene. In theory, the Symbolic father who is the object of the positive transference and the Imaginary father who is the object of Dora's narcissism and her aggressivity are distinguishable. Nevertheless, Dora's father is kept "*hors scène*" by arbitrarily cutting the associative chains that lead to the father and implicate him in the case, by minimizing his role in determining Dora's attitude toward her analyst, and by ignoring the fact that, despite his disclaimers, Freud does in several instances act as his representative—most notably with respect to his portrayal of Dora's mother. If Dora's father must be thus excluded from the scene, it can only be because his entry into it would threaten the schematization that is its principal support: not by showing that the Symbolic order is subject to the Imaginary, not by showing that the Imaginary is charged with Symbolic significance, but by revealing the fundamental complicity of these two orders, their determination in and by the *one* scene.

Lacan's interpretation of *Dora* is ultimately an attempt to reduce the relationships described in the case to the structure of the scene that Irigaray points to as the fundamental scene of psychoanalysis: to the triad little girl/little boy/analyst. Or rather, to an opposition little girl/little boy, and to a synthesis, (the position of) the analyst. But that the phenomenon of countertransference extends to Freud's relation to Dora's father and to Dora herself, as well as to Herr K., means that the dialectical hierarchy within which *Dora* becomes the matrix for the emergence of a psychoanalytic truth is itself determined by a process of doubling.[9] It is this process that constitutes the relationships of *Dora* and that ultimately threatens the originality of the interpretative scene itself. It is this endless process of identification that preempts and predetermines any value, however formal, that might serve as the basis either of a positive transference or of a catharsis effected by a unique identification with a hero—even an absent one.

The countertransference implicates Freud in the scene of psychoanalysis—but not only where Lacan "wants" him to be implicated. By the same token, Lacan's use of procedures "borrowed" from the *Phenomenology* implicates his interpretation of *Dora* in the history of philosophy, but not only in the way he wants it to. The relationship between Hegel and Freud is subject to the same process of doubling as the relationship between Herr K. and Dora's father, and Lacan's interpretations of each relationship hinge on similar strategies. The importation of the Hegelian dialectic into the case study is responsible for the creation of certain interpretative effects—the schematization of the contradictory elements of Dora and a neutralization of the "reversal of the *beautiful soul*" that opens the analysis—and these effects in turn permit the neutralization of Freud's relation to the history of philosophy in general and to Hegel in particular. Like the relationships narrated in *Dora,* the relationship between Hegel and Freud will be "reduced" to a triadic structure composed of a couple (Hegel and the Freud of the countertransference) and a transcendent term (the Freud of the transference). Although, for Lacan, the place designated by Freud's name is empty, it nonetheless comports all the guarantees of the formal coherence of the work that the classical subject does. It is only in the name of such a subject that Lacan can claim to synthesize the conflicts left unresolved by the case and, in so doing, to unveil the truth of *Dora*.

Thus it is not out of fidelity to any truth of Freud or his work that I have traced the *mise en scène* of the problems of (counter) transference and bisexuality to the point at which no synthesis of these two themes is possible. The conflict between them—and *Dora* itself—can no longer be innocently assigned a place in a dialectic that would guarantee their synthesis, nor can it be reduced in the name of a totality that, as the tool of a critical strategy, would itself escape criticism. Even after the death of Freud, a "return to Freud" will not reveal only one Freud and one scene of sexual difference. Insofar as the themes of bisexuality and transference cannot be brought into play without fundamentally implicating psychoanalysis in a whole history whose sense it cannot neutralize, insofar as the handling of these themes cannot but reveal the derivation of the scene of psychoanalysis with respect to a series of conflicts that both define and put into question its limits, *Dora* can only reopen the questions concerning sexuality and Freud's understanding of it that the "return to Freud" has tended to close, and that, in fact, it too reopens.

Notes

1. Sigmund Freud, *The Origins of Psychoanalysis: Sigmund Freud's Letters to Wilhelm Fliess (1887–1902)*, Marie Bonaparte, Anna Freud, and Ernst Kris, eds. (New York: Basic Books, 1954), pp. 215–216.

2. "When a patient brings forward a sound and incontestable train of argument during the psychoanalytic treatment, the physician is liable to feel a moment's embarrassment, and the patient may take advantage of it by asking: 'This is all perfectly true and correct, isn't it? . . .' But it soon becomes evident that the patient is using thoughts of this kind, which the analysis cannot attack, for the purpose of cloaking others that are anxious to escape from criticism and consciousness." *SE* 7:35; *C* 51.

3. Jacques Lacan, *Ecrits* (Paris: Seuil, 1966), p. 221 (Rose, *p. 98*). Gearhart makes her own translations. Unless otherwise specified, page references in text will be to *Ecrits*. For the reader's convenience we have provided cross-references to Jacqueline Rose's translation of "Intervention sur le transfert," essay 4 of this book. Page numbers of the Rose translation will be in italics—Editors' note.

4. Though historically speaking the feminine role is, for Freud, generally played by the little girl, the ultimate significance of the discovery of her "castration" lies in the application of that discovery to the mother. For Luce Irigaray, that the little girl should figure in the scene only as the representative of the mother is itself significant, for according to her analysis, it is the equation of feminine sexuality with maternity that permits Freud to avoid raising the question of feminine sexuality per se and to assimilate it to a fundamentally masculine model in which the child functions as a penis and the desire for a child becomes the woman's dominant sexual aim. Freud's portrayal of what he calls the primary virility of the little girl and the displaced virility of the mother reflects the fundamentally masculine character of desire as it has been defined by psychoanalysis (and not only by psychoanalysis). In this respect, Freud's comments on a young lesbian are of general significance: "A woman who has felt herself to be a man and has loved in a masculine fashion, will hardly let herself

be forced into playing the part of a woman [if] she must pay for this transformation, which is not in every way advantageous, by renouncing all hope of motherhood."

5. Under certain historical and cultural conditions this imaginary relationship to castration can become a norm. Indeed, for Lacan, the normative (ideological) use of psychoanalysis—which he attacks in the form of American ego psychology—represents a reinforcement of the Imaginary.

6. The opposition between the Symbolic and the Imaginary is often supplemented by a third term: the real. But for Lacan, the "real" is not an autonomous term, but rather always a function of one or the other of the two orders (p. 68). That is, the real functions either symbolically, as the impossible, as absence, as a *béance*, or as a projection or mirage of the imaginary values of the *moi*.

7. His interpretation of this scene differs significantly from that proposed by Catherine Clément and Hélène Cixous in *La jeune née* (Paris: 10/18, 1975). For them the slap with which Dora greets Herr K.'s proposition (or proposal) stems directly from her identification with Frau K. and signifies her refusal to accept the contempt for Frau K. (and ultimately for herself as a woman) implicit in Herr K.'s opening words: "You know I get nothing from my wife." Lacan's interpretation takes account of Dora's identification with Herr K. as well as of her identification with Frau K., and Dora's ensuant neuralgia of the cheek supports his interpretation—it is as though she gave and received the slap at the same time.

8. This in itself seems to cast doubt on Lacan's contention, since the *Three Introductory Lectures* and *Dora* appeared in the same year.

9. Freud himself investigated this phenomenon of doubling in the essay that has been translated into English as "The Uncanny." That Freud should thus explicitly thematize this problem puts into question more than the homogeneity of his work; it puts into question the coherence ascribed to it by Lacan and Irigaray. The effects of the process of doubling—the *Unheimlichkeit*—play a central role in Jacques Derrida's fundamental and indispensable reading of psychoanalysis in "Le facteur de la vérité," *Poétique* (1975), no. 21; translated in *Yale French Studies*, no. 52.

6. Dora: Fragment of an Analysis

JACQUELINE ROSE

The word is understood only as an extension of the body which is there in the process of speaking. . . . To the extent that it does not know repression, femininity is the downfall of interpretation.

Michèle Montrelay, "Inquiry Into Femininity," *m/f*, no. 1, p. 89

Filmed sequence—it is the body of Dora which speaks pain, desire, speaks a force divided and contained.

Hélène Cixous, *Portrait de Dora* (Paris, 1976), p. 36

What would it mean to reopen the case of Dora now? The quotations above point to an urgency that is nothing less than that of the present dialogue between psychoanalysis and feminism, a dialogue that seems crucial and yet constantly slides away from the point of a possible encounter, psychoanalysis attempting to delimit an area that might be called femininity within the confines of the drive, within a theory of sexuality that constantly places and displaces the concept of sexual difference, feminism starting precisely from that difference which it then addresses to psychoanalysis as a demand, the demand for the theory of its construction. Feminism, therefore, first turns to psychoanalysis because it is seen as the best place to describe the coming into being of femininity, which, in a next stage, it can be accused of pro-

This essay was first published in *m/f* (1978), no. 2, pp. 5–21.

ducing or at least reproducing, sanctioning somehow within its own discourse. And then, where it fails, as it did with Dora, this can be taken as the sign of the impossibility of its own project, the impossibility then becoming the feminine, which, by a twist that turns the language of psychoanalysis against itself, it *represses.* Quite simply, the case of Dora is seen to fail because Dora is repressed as a woman by psychoanalysis and what is left of Dora as somehow retrievable is the insistence of the body as feminine, and since it is a case of hysteria, in which the symptom speaks across the body itself, the feminine is placed not only as source (origin and exclusion) but also as manifestation (the symptom). Within this definition, hysteria is assimilated to a body as site of the feminine, outside discourse, silent finally, or, at best, "dancing."

What I want to do in this article is look at some of these difficulties through the case of Dora—not simply to accuse the case of its failure, which failure must, however, be described and interrogated; not to produce an alternative reading whose content would be the feminine; but nonetheless to bring out some of the problems of the case precisely as the problem of the feminine within psychoanalysis in its urgency for us now. To do this will involve a discussion of the case itself, how its failure relates to changes in the concept of sexuality, and how these changes, which come at least partly in response to that failure, make certain conceptions of the feminine problematic.

The article falls into three parts: (1) the failure of the case, its relation to Freud's concept of femininity; (2) the relation of changes in the concept of femininity to changes in that of analytic practice (transference), and then to the concept of the unconscious in its relation to representation (hysterical and schizophrenic language); and (3) how these changes make impossible any notion of the feminine that would be outside representation,[1] the failure of the case of Dora being precisely the failure to articulate the relation between these two terms.

THE CASE OF DORA

The case of Dora was first drafted under the title "Dreams and Hysteria" in 1901, the year after the publication of *The Interpretation of*

Dreams. Yet it did not appear until 1905, in the same year as the *Three Essays on a Theory of Sexuality*. The space between the two dates is punctuated by Freud's own comments on his hesitancy regarding a case that had promised so much, that he had in fact promised as nothing less than the sequel to *The Interpretation of Dreams*, as the link between clinical practice and dream analysis, between the etiology of the symptom and the primary process. The history of the case, its hesitancy, in this sense speaks for itself, for it is caught quite literally between those two aspects of Freud's work, the theory of the unconscious and the theory of sexuality, whose relation or distance is what still concerns us today, as if the case of Dora could only appear finally at the point where the implications of its failure had already been displaced onto a theory of sexuality, by no means complete and still highly problematic, but at least acknowledged as such. Dora then falls, or fails, in the space between these two texts, and Freud himself writes: "While the case history before us seems particularly favoured as regards the utilization of dreams, in other respects, it has turned out poorer than I could have wished" (*SE* 7:11; *P* 40; *C* 26).

What then was wrong with Dora? First, in the simple sense of diagnosis and/or symptom, leaving aside at this stage the question of the status of the diagnostic category itself, not forgetting however that it was from this very question that psychoanalysis set out (rejection of hysteria as an independent clinical entity[2]), Dora, then, as first presented or brought to Freud, was suffering from *tussis nervosa* and periodic attacks of aphonia (nervous cough and loss of voice), "possibly migraines, together with depression, hysterical unsociability, and a *taedium vitae* which was probably not entirely genuine." Her entering into the treatment had been precipitated by the discovery of a suicide note by her parents and a momentary loss of consciousness after a row with her father, subsequently covered by amnesia. The symptoms are so slight, in a sense, that Freud feels it necessary to excuse to the reader the attention he is to give to the case, its status as it were as exemplary of a neurotic disorder whose etiology he sets himself to describe.

The situation is all the more complex in that the case is offered as a "fragment," and this in a number of different senses: first, the case was broken off by the patient; second, it was not committed to writing until after the completion of the treatment (only the words of the dreams were recorded immediately after the session); and third, as a corollary to the second factor, only the results of the analysis and not its process were transcribed. Finally, Freud explicitly states that, where the etiology of the case stalled, he appeals to other cases to fill in the gaps, always indicating the point at which "the authentic part ends and my construction begins."

Each of these notions of fragment are crucial for the case, and each is double-edged. If the case is broken off after three months, this only "fragments" it insofar as the whole practice of psychoanalysis had changed from the immediate analysis of the symptom to an engagement with whatever presented itself to the mind of the patient in any one session, so that the inadequacy of the time span is the consequence of a new privileging of the discourse of the patient herself. Thus the distinction between the results and the process of analysis, which is the basis of the second and third notions of fragment, in one sense collapses on the first (this incidentally should be remembered in any simple dismissal of the case as the suppression of the patient's "own" language). On the other hand, the process *is* missing from the case in another and more crucial sense, that of the relation between the analyst and the patient, which Freud calls the transference, and to whose neglect he partly ascribes its failure. All these points should be borne in mind as the signs of this failure, and yet each is a paradox: the process is there, but it is somehow elided; a meaning or interpretation of Dora's "complaint" is produced, but it is clearly inadequate.

To give a history of the case is therefore impossible, but a number of central points can be disengaged that I hope will be of help in the discussion to follow:[3]

1. The parameters of the case are defined by the sexual circuit that runs between Dora's parents and their "intimate" friends, Herr and Frau K., in which Dora herself is caught.
2. Thus, Dora is courted by Herr K., and the crisis that leads to the treatment is partly precipitated by an attempted seduction on his part, which she repudiates.
3. Behind this is the affair between Dora's father and Frau K.; behind this, crucially, the absence of Dora's mother in her relationship both to Dora

("unfriendly"—*SE* 7:20; *P* 50; *C* 35) and to Dora's father (hence his relationship with Frau K.).

4. Behind this again, there is an intimacy which is first that between the two families but which also completes the sexual circuit between them—the intimacy of Dora and Frau K., whose precise content is never given and that functions exactly as the "secret" of the case, the source of the sexual knowledge that Dora undoubtedly has, and that thus cuts straight across from the "manifest" behavior of the participants to the "latent" etiology of the symptoms (Freud's theory of hysteria).

Put at its most crude, Freud's interpretation of the case is based on a simple identification of the oedipal triangle, and starts with Dora's protest at her place in the relationship between Frau K. and her father, that is, with Dora as a pawn who is proferred to Herr K. Thus her repudiation of the latter is the inevitable consequence of an outrage that takes Herr K. as its immediate object, and yet behind which is the figure of the father, who is the object of real reproach. In this way Dora's rejection of Herr K., "still quite young and of prepossessing appearance" (sic) (*SE* 7:29 *n.*3; *P* 60; *C* 44, *n.*15) can be seen as simultaneously oedipal *and* hysterical (repudiation of her own desire). Dora's own desire is defined here as unproblematic—heterosexual and genital. At this stage Freud was still bound to the traumatic theory of neurosis, and he thus traces the repudiation on the part of Dora to an attempted embrace by Herr K. when she was fourteen, which was also repulsed—"the behaviour of this child of fourteen was already entirely and completely hysterical" (*SE* 7:28; *P* 59; *C* 44). To be more precise, therefore, we would have to say that the oedipal triangle is there in the case history but that it is held off by this notion of trauma, which makes of Herr K. the first repudiated object (the seducer). In his analysis of Dora's first dream, there is no doubt that Freud interprets it as a summoning up of an infantile affection for the father *secondarily,* as a defense against Dora's persistent and unquestioned desire for Herr K. (The second dream is then interpreted as revealing the vengeance/hostility against her father that could not achieve expression in the first.)

Now the way in which the case history is laid out immediately spoils the picture, or the "fine poetic conflict" (*SE* 7:59; *P* 94; *C* 77) as Freud himself puts it, since Dora has been totally complicit in the affair between her father and Frau K., and it had in fact been entirely through her complicity that the situation had been able to continue. Furthermore, Dora's symptom, her cough, reveals an unmistakable identification with her father, a masculine identification confirmed by the appearance of her brother at three points in the case history—each time as the object of identification, whether as recollection, screen memory, or manifest content of the dream. The revealing of this masculine identification leads directly to the uncovering of the "true" object of Dora's jealousy (made clear if for no other reason by the overinsistence of her reproaches against her father), that is, Frau K. herself, with whom Dora had shared such intimacy, secrecy, and confessions, even about Frau K.'s unsatisfactory relationship with her husband, in which case, Freud asks, how on earth could Dora in fact be in love with Herr K.? We may well ask.

What we therefore have in the case is a series of contradictions, which Freud then attempts to resolve by a mandatory appeal to the properties of the unconscious itself ("in the unconscious contradictory thoughts live very comfortably side by side"—*SE* 7:61; *P* 96; *C* 79) revealing a theory of interpretation actually functioning as "resistance" to the pressing need to develop a theory of sexuality, whose complexity or difficulty manifests itself time and again in the case. Thus in his analysis of the hysterical symptom—aphonia, or loss of voice—Freud is forced toward the beginnings of a concept of component sexuality (a sexuality multiple and fragmented and not bound to the genital function), since the symptom is clearly not only the response to the absence of Herr K. (impossibility of the communication desired) but also a fantasied identification with a scene of imagined sexual satisfaction between Dora's father and Frau K. This is the fullest discussion of sexuality in the book, which anticipates many of the theses of the *Three Essays,* but it is conducted by Freud as an apology for Dora (and himself)—justification of the discussion of sexual matters with a young girl (the question therefore being that of censorship, Freud's discovery reduced to the articulation of sexuality *to* a woman) and then as insistence on the perverse and undifferentiated nature of infantile sexuality so that Dora's envisaging of a scene of oral gratification, for that is what it is, might be less of a scandal.

The difficulties therefore clearly relate to the whole concept of sexuality, and not just to the nature of the object (for the importance of this, see later in this essay on the concept of the sexual aim), but Freud's own resistance appears most strongly in relation to Frau K.'s status as an object of desire for Dora. Thus this aspect of the case surfaces only symptomatically in the text, at the end of the clinical picture that it closes, and in a series of footnotes and additions to the interpretation of the second dream and in the postscript.

It is in her second dream that the identification of Dora with a man (her own suitor) is unquestionable, and since the analysis reveals a latent obsession with the body of the woman, the Madonna, defloration, and finally childbirth, the recuperation of a primary autoeroticism (the masturbation discerned behind the first dream) by a masculine fantasy of self-possession now charted across the question of sexual difference is clear.[4] Yet Freud makes of the dream an act of vengeance, as he does the breaking off of the case, which perhaps not surprisingly is its immediate sequel. The way this dream raises the question of sexual difference will be discussed below. It should already serve as a caution against any assimilation of Dora's homosexual desire for Frau K. to a simple preoedipal instance. Note for the moment that Freud is so keen to hang onto a notion of genital heterosexuality that it leads him, first, to identify the fantasy of childbirth that analysis revealed behind the second dream as an "obscure maternal longing" (*SE* 7:104, *n.*2; *P* 145; *C* 125, *n.*20), outdoing in advance Karen Horney's appeals to such a longing as natural, biological and pregiven, in her attacks on Freud's later work on femininity, and second, to classify Dora's masculine identification and desire for Frau K. as "gynaecophilic" and to make it "typical of the unconscious erotic life of hysterical girls" (*SE* 7:63; *P* 98; *C* 81), that is, to use as an explanation of hysteria the very factor that needs to be explained.

Finally, it should be pointed out that the insistence on a normal genital sexuality is obviously related to the question of transference. Freud himself attributes the failure of the case to his failure in "mastering the transference in good time" (*SE* 7:118; *P* 160; *C* 140), while his constant footnoting of this discussion with references to his overlooking the homosexual desire of his patient indicates that the relation between these two aspects of the case remains unformulated. At one level it is easy to see that Freud's failure to understand his own implication in the case (countertransference) produced a certain definition of sexuality as a *demand* on Dora, which, it should be noted, she rejects (walks out). On the other hand, and more crucially, Freud's own definition of transference in its relation to the cure can be seen as caught in the same trap as that of his theory of sexuality, since he sees the former as the obstacle to the uncovering of "new memories, dealing, probably, with actual events" (*SE* 7:119; *P* 160; *C* 141) (relics of the seduction theory), just as he defines neurosis as the failure "to meet a real erotic demand" (*SE* 7:110; *P* 151; *C* 132), and even allows (thereby undermining the whole discovery of psychoanalysis) that neurosis might ultimately be vanquished by "reality" (*SE* 7:110; *P* 152; *C* 132). The concept of a possible recovery from neurosis through reality and that of an unproblematic feminine sexuality are coincident in the case.

"IN FACT SHE WAS A FEMINIST"

The reference comes from Freud's case on the "Psychogenesis of Homosexuality in a Woman," and in one sense the step from the failure of the case of Dora to this case, which appeared in 1920, is irresistible—not, however, in order to classify Dora as homosexual in any simple sense, but precisely because in this case Freud was led to an acknowledgment of the homosexual factor in all feminine sexuality, an acknowledgment which was to lead to his revision of his theories of the Oedipus complex for the girl. For in this article he is in a way at his most radical, rejecting the concept of cure, insisting that the most psychoanalysis can do is restore the original bisexual disposition of the patient, defining homosexuality as nonneurotic. Yet, at the same time, his explanation of this last factor—the lack of neurosis ascribed to the fact that the object-choice was established not in infancy but after puberty—is then undermined by his being obliged to trace back the homosexual attraction to a moment prior to the oedipal instance, the early attachment to the mother, in which case either the girl is neurotic (which she clearly is not) or all women are neurotic (which indeed they might be).

The temptation is therefore to see the case of Dora as anticipating, through the insistence of Dora's desire for Frau K. as substitute for the absent mother in the case ("the mystery turns upon your mother," Freud says in relation to the first dream—*SE* 7:70; *P* 105; *C* 87), the nature of the preoedipal attachment between mother and girl child, an attachment Freud finally makes specific to feminine sexuality in its persistence and difficulty. All recent work on the concept of a feminine sexuality that resists or exceeds the reproductive or genital function stems from this, and since the Oedipus complex is properly the insertion of the woman into the circuit of symbolic exchange (nothing could be clearer in the case of Dora), then her resistance to this positioning is assigned a radical status. The woman, therefore, is outside exchange, an exchange put into play or sanctioned by nothing other than language itself, which thus produces the question of her place and *her* language simultaneously. The transition to a concept of hysterical discourse as some privileged relation to the maternal body is then easy; it is partly supported by Freud's own "suspicion" that "this phase of attachment to the mother is especially intimately related to the etiology of hysteria, which is not surprising when we reflect that both the phase and the neurosis are characteristically feminine" ("Female Sexuality," *SE* 21:227).

What seems to happen is that the desire to validate the preoedipal instance as resistance to the oedipal structure itself leads to a "materialization" of the *bodily* relation that underpins it, so that the body of the mother, or more properly the girl's relation to it, is then placed as being somehow outside repression. What we then have is a constant assimilation in feminist texts of the maternal body and the unrepressed (see Montrelay, quoted at the beginning of this article), or of the maternal body and the dream (Kristeva: "different, close to the dream or the maternal body"), or of the maternal body and a primary autoeroticism (Irigaray) whose return would apparently mean the return of the (feminine) exile.[5] In the case of Kristeva, the relation to differing modes of language is made explicit to the point of identifying a preoedipal linguistic register (rhythms, intonations) and a postoedipal linguistic register (the phonologico-syntactic structure of the sentence). Hysteria, therefore, and the poetic language of the woman (which becomes the language of women poets, Woolf, Plath, etc.) are properly then the return of this primary and bodily mode of expressivity.[6] It is no coincidence that at this stage it is schizophrenia that is invoked as frequently as hysteria, since the relation between schizophrenia and poetic discourse is a recognized and accredited one within psychoanalysis itself. It is in a sense a feminist version of Laing, but having to include the transference neurosis (hysteria) since the relation of the latter to the feminine is too heavily attested to be ignored. More often than not, the two forms are assimilated the one to the other, so that what happens is that the specificity of the two types of disorder is lost. It is worth, therefore, looking again at Dora's symptoms, and then (in the next section) at what Freud said about schizophrenia in its relation to language, in order to see whether such a position can be theoretically sustained.

A number of points about Dora first. First, as we saw above, Dora's bodily symptoms (the aphonia, the cough) are the expression of a masculine identification, through which identification alone access to the maternal and feminine body is possible. This access then threatens Dora with a physical or bodily fragmentation, which constitutes the symptoms of conversion. Thus access to the (maternal) body is only possible now through a masculine identification, which access then threatens the very category of identification itself, that is, Dora as subject. Thus at neither point of her desire for Frau K. can Dora be placed as a "true" feminine, since either she is identified with a man or else the movement is toward an instance in which the category of sexual difference is not established and that of the subject, on which such difference depends, is threatened.

Second, in the second dream, in which Dora's desire could be defined as the desire for self-possession, her position as subject is at its most precarious. The dream most clearly articulates the split between the subject and object of enunciation at the root of any linguistic utterance (the speaking subject and the subject of the statement),[7] here seen in its relation to the question of sexual difference. Thus, if Dora is there to be possessed, then she is not there as a woman (she is a man), and if she is not there to be possessed, her place as a woman is assured (she remains feminine) but she is not there (Lacan's lethal *vel*).[8]

Third, and as a corollary to this, what is revealed behind this dream is nothing other than this question of woman *as* representation: "Here for the third time we come upon 'picture' (views of towns, the Dresden gallery), but in a much more significant connection. Because of what appears in the picture (the wood, the nymphs), the 'Bild' (picture) is turned into a 'Weibsbild' (literally 'picture of a woman')" (*SE* 7:99, *n.*1; *P* 139; *C* 119, *n.*11), and then of woman *as* query, posed by Dora herself, of her relationship to a knowledge designated as present and not present—the sexual knowledge that is the *secret* behind her relation with Frau K.: "Her *knowing* all about such things and, at the same time, her *pretending not to know where her knowledge came from* was really too remarkable. I ought to have attacked this *riddle* and looked for the motive of such a remarkable piece of repression" (*SE* 7:120, *n.*1; *P* 162; *C* 142, *n.*2; italics mine). Thus nothing in Dora's position can be assimilated to an unproblematic concept of the feminine or to any simple notion of the body, since where desire is genital it is charted across a masculine identification, and where it is oral it reveals itself as a query addressed to the category of sexuality itself (Frau K. as the "unmistakable *oral* source of information" (*SE* 7:105, *n.*2; *P* 145; *C* 126, *n.*20).[9]

Perhaps we should remember here that Freud's work on hysteria started precisely with a rejection of any simple mapping of the symptom onto the body (Charcot's hysterogenic zones). By so doing he made of hysteria a language (made it speak) but one whose relation to the body was decentered, since if the body spoke it was precisely because there was something called the unconscious that could not. At this point the relation of dreams and hysteria, from which we started out, can be reasserted as nothing other than the inflection of the body *through* language in its relation to the unconscious (indirect representation). When Lacan writes that "there is nothing in the unconscious with which the body accords" he means this, and he continues: "The unconscious is discordant. The unconscious is that which, by speaking, determines the subject as being, but a being to be struck through with that metonymy by which I support desire insofar as it is endlessly impossible to speak as such."[10] We saw this above in the split between subject and object of enunciation, Dora as subject literally fading before her presence in the dream.

WORD-PRESENTATIONS AND THING-PRESENTATIONS

Freud's discussion of schizophrenic and hysterical language is at its most explicit in chapter 7 of his metapsychological paper on the unconscious (*SE* 14:196–205). That this discussion should take up the chapter entitled "Assessment of the Unconscious" indicates its importance, and it is in fact the distinction between these two types of disorder that produces Freud's definition of the concept UCS (the unconscious in his system: unconscious, preconscious, and conscious). Freud starts with schizophrenia in its inaccessibility to analysis, involving as it does a complete withdrawal of object-cathexes in their reversion to the ego. Note that what this produces is unmitigated narcissism, so that while the definition indicates Freud still basing his diagnostic categories on a differential relation to reality, what emerges at another level is a concept of schizophrenia as the "embodiment" of the category of the ego and hence of identification (as opposed to the embodiment of the body). What then appears as symptom is what Freud calls organ-speech, in which "the patient's relation to the bodily organ [arrogates] to itself the representation of the whole content [of her thoughts]." Thus the precondition of organ-speech is a reversion to narcissism, and the function of the body is the representation of a thought-content, which, in both of the examples given, reveals the patient's identification with her lover; this as distinct from the hysterical symptom, where there is not the verbal articulation of a certain relation to the body but the bodily symptom itself, i.e., conversion.

Hence there can be no equating of schizophrenia and hysteria and no assimilation of either to the body in an unmediated form. On the other hand, if the attempt to construct a theory of feminine discourse tends to produce such an identification, it is because of the attraction for such a theory of what Freud says about the schizophrenic's privileged relation to words (subject to the primary processes and obeying the laws of the unconscious) and the definition that this then leads to of unconscious representation itself: "We now seem to know all at once what the difference is between conscious and unconscious presentation—the conscious presentation comprises the presentation of the thing and the presentation of the word, while the unconscious presentation is the presentation of the thing alone" (*SE* 14:201). The distinction does in fact appear to be predicated on the notion of some direct, ("truer" even) relation to the object itself: "The system UCS contains the thing-cathexes of the objects, the first and true object-cathexes" (*SE* 14:201).

It is on the collapse of this concept, in Freud's text itself, that the assimilation schizophrenia/body/unconscious can again be seen to fail. First, Freud does in fact state even within this definition that what is involved in the first (primary) cathexis of the object is the memory-*trace* of the object, and in the appendix on aphasia he states the relation between object and thing-presentation to be a mediate one. Second, in the choice that his distinction leaves him—for if the unconscious comprises the thing-presentation alone, repression involving a withdrawal of the word, then for the schizophrenic either there is no repression or else the schizophrenic's use of language indicates the first stage of a *recovery,* the recovery of the object-cathexes themselves. The schizophrenic's relation to the word would therefore reveal at its most transparent the loss of the object that is at the root of linguistic representation ("These endeavours are directed towards *regaining the lost object*"—*SE* 14:204). This is the concept at the basis of the concept of the unconscious as the *effect* of the subject's insertion into language, the loss of the object and production of the subject in that moment (the moment of its fading).

A number of conceptions about language that underpin discussion about the feminine and discourse, the feminine *as* discourse can now be disengaged. First, the idea of an unmediated relation between the body and language is contrary to the linguistic definition of the sign, implying as it does a type of anatomical mimesis of language on the body (for example, Irigaray's "two lips" as indicating the place of woman outside (phallo-)monistic discourse). Second, the concept of the feminine as outside discourse involves a theory of language in which a nonexcentric relation to language would be possible, the subject as control and origin of meaning, which is to render meaningless both the concept of the unconscious and that of the subject.

It is on this latter factor that the relation of psychoanalysis to language exceeds that of linguistics, precisely insofar as it poses this problem of the subject's relation to discourse. Freud did not formulate this as such, but it is there in the contradictions of his text, in this further sense, too, and most clearly, I would suggest, in what he has to say about feminine sexuality and transference—which brings us back to the case of Dora.

THE QUESTION OF FEMININITY

In this final section I want to look at the two "vanishing points" of the case of Dora—the theory of feminine sexuality and the concept of transference. For if the case failed it was because Freud failed to recognize the specificity of either of these two factors, and where he saw their pertinence (addenda, postscript, footnote) they were left in a type of offstage of the case, as the thing that was missing (the "secret") or the element that he had failed to "master," as if both were a content, an object to be identified, placed, and resolved (transference as the recovery of an actual event). What I want to do here, therefore, is to show how in both of these concepts something of the subject's relation to discourse as we saw it emerging above—in Dora's second dream, and then in the schizophrenic relation to the word—can be discerned and to suggest the pertinence of that theory for discussion of the feminine not *as* discourse but, within discourse, as a relationship to it.

First, the transference, as it was elaborated by Freud in his papers on technique ("The Dynamics of Transference," "Remembering, Repeating, and Working-Through," "Observations on the Transference-Love"), where he starts again with a definition of neurosis as a libidinal turning away from reality, is first seen as a resistance in the chain of associations that would lead logically to the repairing or completing of the patient's memory. Dora's case also started, in Freud's discussion of the fragment, with this insistence that cure of the symptom and completion of memory were synonymous—psychoanalysis defined here as the creation of a full history to which the subject would be restored. It is a concept also present at the beginning of Lacan's work on the idea of full speech,[11] retranscription of the history of the patient *through* language, before the development of the concept of the unconscious precisely as the effect *of* language, and hence behind it a moment of failing that can never be restored, that is nothing other than that of the subject itself (primary repression). Thus Freud starts by stressing transference as the obstacle to the reality of the patient's history, in a simple sense corresponding to the notion that behind neurosis is an event (seduction theory) and in front of it, if all goes well, another event (neurosis vanquished by reality), transference appearing here as something that "flings" the patient "out of his real relation to the doctor" ("The Dynamics of Transference," *SE* 12:107).

Yet, taken together, these three texts inscribe an opposite movement. In the discussion of recollection ("Remembering, Repeating, and Working-Through"), Freud interpolates a discussion of amnesia that starts with the concept of total recall as the objective of analysis but ends up with a discussion of primary or primal fantasy, indicating that concept of Freud's which was most completely to undermine the concept of the cure as the retrieval of a real occurrence. In fact, in his article on the two principles of mental functioning (*SE* 12:213–227), Freud assigned to fantasy the whole domain of sexuality, whereby it escapes the reality principle altogether (pleasure in sexuality revealing itself as pleasure in the act of representation itself).

Through this a different concept of the transference emerges, one seen most clearly in "Observations on Transference-Love," where what is objected to in transference is its status as a demand (the demand for love) and, more important, one that insists on being recognized as *real* (which it is, Freud has to concede), so that what now "irrupts" into the analytic situation is reality itself, a reality that is totally out of place: "There is a complete change of scene; it is as though some piece of make-believe had been stopped by the sudden irruption of reality" (*SE* 12:162). The patient insists therefore on repeating "in real life" what should only have been reproduced as "psychical material"—thus the relationship to the real has been reversed. What this indicates for this discussion is that Freud himself was forced to correct or to revise the concept of transference to which he ascribed the failure of the case of Dora, and this in a way that is not satisfactorily or exhaustively defined by reference to the countertransference (Freud's implication in the case). For what is at stake is transference as an impossible demand for recognition (a return of love in "Observations on the Transference-Love"), a demand that has to be displaced onto another register, indicated here by the corresponding emphasis on the concepts of fantasy ("make-believe"), representation, psychical material (the only meaning of material that has any value here). Note the proximity of these terms to the query, image, *Bild,* of Dora's second dream, sexuality precisely not as demand (the demand for love) but as question.

In the discussion of the case itself, I suggested that Freud's concept of the transference as the retrieval of an event corresponded to the concept of a pregiven normal feminine sexuality, neurosis being defined as the failure to meet a "real erotic demand." Thus if the concept of reality has to go in relation to the notion of transference, we can reasonably assume that it also goes in relation to that of sexuality itself. I have already suggested briefly that it does, in what Freud says about the pleasure principle. What is important to grasp is that, while it is undoubtedly correct to state that Freud's analysis of Dora failed because of the theory of feminine sexuality to which he then held, this concept cannot be corrected by a simple reference to his later theses on feminine sexuality (preoedipality, etc.), crucial as these may be, since that is simply to replace one content with another, whereas what must be seen in Freud's work on femininity is exactly the same movement we have just seen in the concept of transference, which is nothing less than the collapse of the category of sexuality as *content* altogether.

Freud starts both his papers on femininity ("Female Sexuality" and "Femininity") with recognition of the girl's preoedipal attachment to the mother, its strength and duration, as it had been overlooked within psychoanalytic theory, thus feminine sexuality as an earlier stage, a more repressed content, something archaic. Yet, although the two papers in one sense say the same thing, their logic or sequence is different, and the difference has important effects on the level of theory.

"Female Sexuality" (1931) starts with the preoedipal factor and its necessary relinquishment, which is then discussed in terms of the castration complex and penis envy. But this does not exhaust the question of the girl's renunciation of her mother, a question that then persists in a series of references to "premature" weaning, the advent of a rival, the necessary frustration and final ambivalence of the child's demand for love. None of these factors, however, constitute a sufficient explanation: "All these motives seem nevertheless insufficient to justify the girl's final hostility" (*SE* 21:234), which cannot be attributed to the ambivalence of the infantile relation to the object, since this would be true of the boy child too. Thus a question persists that reveals itself as *the* question, hanging over from that of a demand that has been frustrated and a renunciation that still has not been explained: "A further question arises, 'What does the little girl require of her mother?' " (*SE* 21:235).

Freud can only answer this question by reference to the nature of the infantile sexual aim—its activity (rejection of a male/female biological chemistry, a single libido with both active and passive aims), an activity that is not only a corrective to the idea of a naturally passive femininity but functions as *repetition* (the child repeats a distressing experience through play). Correlating this with the definition of infantile sexuality given earlier in the paper ("It has in point of fact no aim, and is incapable of obtaining complete satisfaction and principally for that reason is doomed to end in disappointment"—*SE* 21:231), it emerges that what specifies the little girl's aim, and her demand, is that she does not have one. The question persists, or is repeated, therefore, as the impossibility of satisfaction.

In "Femininity" (1933), the sequence is in a sense reversed. The paper starts with the caution against the biological definition of sexual difference and then reposes the question of the girl's relinquishment of the preoedipal attachment to the mother. The motives for renunciation are listed again—oral frustration, jealousy, prohibition, ambivalence—but in this case the question of how these can explain such renunciation when they apply equally to the boy is answered with the concept of penis envy, with which the question is in a sense closed (the discussion moves on to a consideration of adult modes of feminine sexuality). Thus the question is answered here, and it is as answer that the concept of penis envy has produced, rightly, the anger against Freud. For looking at the paper again, it is clear that nothing has been answered at all, since Freud characterizes each of the earlier motives specifically in terms of its impossibility (see above): oral demand as "insatiable," "the child's demands for love are immoderate" (rivalry), "multifarious sexual wishes which cannot for the most part be satisfied," "the immoderate character of the demand for love and the impossibility of fulfilling their sexual wishes" (*SE* 22:122, 123, 124). Now, if what characterizes all these demands is the impossibility of their satisfaction, then the fact that there is another impossible demand ("the wish to get the longed-for penis"—*SE* 22:125) cannot strictly explain anything at all, other than the persistence of the demand itself—the question, therefore, of the earlier paper, "What does the little girl require of her mother?"[12]

The question persists, therefore, only insofar as it cannot be answered, and what I want to suggest here is that what we see opening up in the gap between the demand and its impossibility is desire itself, what Lacan calls the effect of the articulation of need as demand, "desire endlessly impossible to speak as such." This is why the demand for love in the transference blocks the passage of the treatment insofar as it insists precisely on its own reality (the possibility of satisfaction). What Freud's papers on femininity reveal, therefore, is nothing less than the emergence of this concept of desire as the *question* of sexual difference: how does the little girl become a woman, or does she?

To return to dreams and hysteria, isn't this exactly the question that reveals itself in the dream of the hysteric analyzed in *The Interpretation of Dreams* (*SE* 4:147–151) who dreamt that her own wish was *not* fulfilled, through an identification with the woman she posited as her sexual rival? Her desire, therefore, is the desire for an unsatisfied desire: "She likes caviar," writes Lacan, "but she doesn't want any. It is in that that she desires it."[13] And behind that wish (and that identification) the question of the woman as object of desire, of how her husband could desire a woman who was incapable of giving him satisfaction (she knows he does not want her), the identification, therefore, with the question itself: "This being the question put forward, which is very generally that of hysterical identification, whereby the woman identifies herself with the man."[14] This can be referred directly back to the case of Dora, woman as object and subject of desire—the impossibility of either position, for if object of desire then whose desire, and if subject of desire then its own impossibility, the impossibility of subject *and* desire (the one implying the fading of the other). Thus Dora rejects Herr K. at the exact moment when he states that he does not desire his own wife, the very woman through whom the whole question for Dora was posed (the scene on the lake).

Thus what feminine sexuality reveals in these examples is the persistence of the question of desire *as* a question (exactly the opposite of the feminine as sexual content, substance, or whatever). Finally, to return to the hysterical symptom itself:

> It is to the extent that a need gets caught up in the function of desire that the psychosomatic can be conceived of as something more than the idle commonplace which consists in saying that there is a psychic backing to everything somatic. That much we have known for a long time. If we speak of the psychosomatic it is insofar as what must intervene is desire.[15]

I want to conclude with this, not because I think it answers anything but because I believe it to be a necessary caution to certain current developments within feminist theory. What seems to me to need attention is precisely this movement of psychoanalysis away from sexuality as content (preoedipal or otherwise) to a concept of sexuality as caught up in the register of demand and desire. What does emerge from the above is that it was on the failings in the concept of the feminine (the case of Dora) that this problem emerged in Freud's own work. To relinquish the idea of a specific feminine discourse may be less discouraging if what it leads to is work on the place of the feminine as somehow revealing more urgently the impossibility of the position of the woman within a discourse that would prefer to suppress the question of desire as such (the question of its splitting). I would suggest that the case of Dora reveals no more, and no less, than this.

Notes

1. See Parveen Adams, "Representation and Sexuality," *m/f* (1978), no. 1.

2. See Breuer and Freud's *Studies on Hysteria, SE* 2.

3. For a fuller discussion of the sequence of this case, see Lacan, "Intervention on Transference," in this volume.

4. Note Freud's discussion of this dream: "What was most evident was that in this first part of the dream she was identifying herself with a young man—it would have been appropriate for the goal to have been the possession of a woman, of herself." *SE* 7:96–97; *P* 136; *C* 116–117.

5. Julia Kristeva, *Des chinoises* (Paris: Editions des femmes, 1974); *About Chinese Women*, Anita Barrows, tr. (New York: Urizen Books, 1977); Luce Irigaray, *Speculum de l'autre femme* (Paris: Minuit, 1974).

6. It can also be objected to these arguments that they simply reproduce the classical definition of women/the feminine as irrational, outside discourse, language, etc., with clearly reactionary implications for women. See, for discussion of this, Monique Plaza, "Pouvoir 'phallomorphique' et psychologie de 'la Femme' " in *Questions feministes*, no. 1 (Paris: Editions tierce, 1977), translated in *Ideology and Consciousness*, no. 4 (1978), as " 'Phallomorphic' Power and the Psychology of 'Women'—A Patriarchal Chain."

7. This is the linguistic distinction between the subject of the enunciation and the subject of the enunciated (Emile Benveniste, "De la subjectivité dans le langage," in *Problèmes de linguistique generale* [Paris: Gallimard, 1966]; trans., University of Miami Press, 1971), which I deliberately reformulate here. For a discussion of the concept for psychoanalysis, see J. Lacan, "Analyse et vérité ou la fermeture de l'inconscient," in *Le Seminaire XI: Les Quatre concepts fondamentaux de la psychanalyse* (Paris: Seuil, 1973); "Analysis and Truth or the Closure of the Unconscious," in *The Four Fundamental Concepts of Psychoanalysis* (New York: Norton, 1978).

8. For a discussion of this, see Parveen Adams, "Representation and Sexuality," p. 72.

9. See Freud's whole footnote here, *SE* 7:104–5, *n.*2; also pp. 110–111, *n.*1 and p. 120, *n.*1 (*P* 145, 152, 162; *C* 125–126, *n.*20, also pp. 132–133, *n.*26, and p. 142, *n.*2).

10. Jacques Lacan, "Séminaire," J.-A. Miller, ed., *Ornicar: Bulletin périodique du champ freudien* (May 1975), no. 3, p. 105. (All translations from Lacan are by Jacqueline Rose).

11. J. Lacan, "Fonction et champ de la parole et du langage en psychanalyse," in *Ecrits* (Paris: Seuil, 1966); "The Function and Field of Speech and Language in Psychoanalysis," in *Ecrits: A Selection* (New York: Norton, 1977).

12. "Feminine Sexuality in Psychoanalytic Doctrine," in Juliet Mitchell and Jacqueline Rose, eds., *Feminine Sexuality: Jacques Lacan and the école freudienne* (New York: Norton, 1983).

13. For a full discussion of this dream, see Jacques Lacan, "La Direction de la cure et les principes de son pouvoir," in *Écrits;* "The Direction of the Treatment and the Principles of its Power," in *Écrits: A Selection.*

14. Lacan, *Ecrits,* p. 126.

15. Jacques Lacan, "Le transfert et la pulsion," "Le champ de l'autre, et retour sur la pulsion," in *Les quatre concepts fondamentaux;* "The Transference and the Drive," "The Field of the Other and Back to the Transference," in *The Four Fundamental Concepts.*

7. Freud's Dora, Dora's Hysteria

MARIA RAMAS

Freud's *Dora* case, formally titled "Fragment of an Analysis of a Case of Hysteria," is one of his best-known case histories. It is read as literary classic, as sociology, as popular romantic fiction and, occasionally perhaps, even as soft core pornography. The Collier paperback, currently in its fifth edition, certainly has been designed to entice a broader audience than psychoanalysts. Its back cover bears the titillating heading, "Dora—her homosexual . . . love for Frau K. was the strongest unconscious current in her mental life." It advertises the cast of supporting characters as "an obsessive mother, an adulterous father,

This essay is a shortened version, edited by the author for this anthology, of an essay that first appeared in *Feminist Studies* (1980), 6:472–510. The full version is reprinted in *Sex and Class in Women's History*, Judith L. Newton, Mary P. Ryan, and Judith R. Walkowitz, eds. (London: Routledge and Kegan Paul, 1983).

I would like to thank Robert Brenner, Shirl Buss, Lynn Fonfa, Stella Menatos, and Victor Wolfenstein for their critical comments on earlier versions of this essay. I would also like to thank Betsy Perry for her helpful suggestions on modifying the article for this publication. In particular, I am indebted to Dawn Baker and Temma Kaplan for countless fascinating and fruitful discussions about *Dora* and about psychoanalysis in general. Of course, the errors are mine alone. The author.

her father's mistress, Frau K., and Frau K.'s husband, who had made amorous advances to Dora."

But "Fragment of an Analysis" is not only romantic fiction. It is considered a classic analysis of the structure and genesis of hysteria and has the first or last word in almost every psychoanalytic discussion of hysteria. Although some have written addenda to Freud's case study, following up on one or another of Dora's multiple identifications or reconsidering the case from the point of view of ego psychology, or from that of technique, or transference, the essential meaning of the analysis remains unchallenged. Dora's frigidity, so haunting to Freud and to us, is still considered a cornerstone of hysteria and its most profound symptom. And the meaning Freud attributed to it is still considered to be "truth" by psychoanalytic theory and by popular culture.[1]

Although psychoanalysts seem to have determined the full meaning of Freud's Dora and Dora's hysteria, I would like to look at this case once again with feminist eyes. My intention is not to use feminism to explain away the unconscious meaning of Dora's hysteria or to deny psychoanalytic discoveries. I will argue, however, that Freud's analysis is only partly true—intriguing fiction and flawed analysis—because it is structured around a fantasy of femininity and female sexuality that remains misunderstood, unconscious if you will. This fantasy continues to be an essential part of psychoanalytic explanations of hysteria, forcing the recognition that psychoanalysis is not simply the theory of the formation of gender identity and sexuality in patriarchal society but is profoundly ideological as well.[2]

At the most obvious and general level, the hysteria of Dora, whose real name was Ida Bauer, signified *refusal,* "negative sexuality," as Steven Marcus calls it. Freud recognized this but never deciphered the meaning of the refusal. While Freud's analysis is complex, his main proposition is a simple one. Freud claimed that Ida Bauer was aroused by Herr K.'s pursuit of her but was unwilling to acknowledge her desire consciously. Her unwillingness, he argued, had many accidental and even healthy motives—for example, "good sense" and "respectability"—but also, importantly, a "neurotic element, namely, the tendency to a repudiation of sexuality which was already present in her"

(*SE* 7:88; *C* 108). Her hysterical symptoms were compromise formations that represented both her desire to yield to Herr K. and a composite force rebelling against that desire. Freud further contended that underlying the present desire for Herr K. was an earlier incestuous childhood wish to be seduced by her father—a wish that she summoned up to protect her from the more recent pressing threat.

I wish to suggest a very different interpretation, however. While reviewing the main evidence for Freud's proposition, I propose to demonstrate that the analysis is not only forced and ultimately unconvincing but that it also begs the question. Ida Bauer's hysteria—her repudiation of sexuality—is not explained by Freud but, rather, explained away; for in the course of the analysis, Freud abandons his initial concern—the elucidation of hysteria as a *compromise formation*—in order to develop an argument that is fundamentally an ideological construct, a construct that defends patriarchal fantasies of femininity and female sexuality.

By engaging in a critical dialogue with Freud's case history, I hope to offer the beginnings of a more cogent explanation for Ida Bauer's *refusal.* Proceeding from a general theoretical to an historically specific level of analysis, I will argue that at the deepest level of meaning, Ida Bauer's hysteria was exactly what it appeared to be—a repudiation of the meaning of heterosexuality. Drawing upon psychoanalytic insight, I will contend that the elementary structures within which female heterosexuality and patriarchal femininity are negotiated pose barriers to their development. These barriers can be schematically viewed as twofold. First, because sexuality is not given but *created* through activity, and because it is created in relation to a woman and the female body, its transfer to a male "object" is problematic. Second, because the essential social relations between men and women are structured in terms of dominance and submission, sexual union is understood accurately as a power relation. In sexual fantasy, this conception takes the form of what psychoanalysis terms "primal scene" fantasies. These fantasies are sadomasochistic in content and have rigidly defined masculine and feminine positions. They are, perhaps, the most profound ideology precisely because they are eroticized. These fantasies take shape at the oedipal "moment" and are intimately bound up with the process by which the child confronts and comes to terms with the patriarchal meanings of sexual difference.

Drawing upon historical evidence, and upon Ida Bauer's personal history as Freud revealed it, I will then explore the specific ways in which these contradictions were posed to Ida Bauer. I will argue that Ida Bauer's hysteria represented a nonresolution of these contradictions and that her hysteria appears for this reason to be a compromise formation. On the one hand, as Freud of course argues, Ida's hysteria revealed attempts to comply with the patriarchal laws of her culture and to appropriate patriarchal femininity and sexuality. This is most clearly revealed in her relationship to Herr K. and in her hysterical identification with servant women. On the other hand, however, her hysteria represented a revolt against this attempt to comply, and it is precisely the forcefulness of this revolt that reveals the brittle and really superficial nature of her compliance. It is this rebellion, unconscious and therefore ineffectual, that must be understood.

I will also contend that Ida Bauer's hysteria, insofar as it expressed a wish, sought to preserve preoedipal love for the mother/woman and to retain access to the maternal/female body. This wish underlay Ida Bauer's identifications with masculinity and her primary focus on oral sexuality. Insofar as her hysteria was denial, it was a repudiation not only of the feminine position in the "primal scene," and the subordination it implied, but a continual, unsuccessful attempt to repudiate the "scene" itself and the sadistic meaning of the phallus. It was an attempt to deny patriarchal sexuality, and it was a protest against postoedipal femininity.

CONTRADICTIONS

In 1897, three years before Ida Bauer's analysis, Freud wrote to Wilhelm Fliess that he had discovered the Oedipus complex, the crucible in which a disparate, infantile sexuality is organized as masculine and feminine and out of which a gendered personality emerges (*SE* 1:265). For the boy, the incestuous desire for the mother is shattered by the recognition of the Father's Law, which prohibits incest, and the Father's punishment for transgressing the Law: castration. At this moment of the discovery of the Father-as-castrator, a childhood theory about the origins of sexual difference is transposed to another register to become the primal fantasy of castration. It is a stark crystallization of the dominant social meaning of sexual difference in patriarchal culture. And while we do not wish to reduce this fantasy in any simple way to material reality, neither can we sever it from an historically developed ensemble of social relations that ultimately, and in a variety of ways, presents masculinity as an infinitely more desirable alternative than femininity.

Freud's original concept of the Oedipus complex, and subsequent reformulations, were developed on the model of the little boy. The theoretical problem of the feminine Oedipus complex was not considered until over a quarter of a century after "Fragment of an Analysis" was written. When Freud finally did consider the issue, he found himself confronting a provocative problem. Both sexes, he realized, must enter the Oedipus complex incestuously desiring the mother. For, while Freudian theory posits a preoedipal child with a polymorphously perverse sexuality, directing passive and active desires toward both parents, the tendency is for the mother to assume primary importance because of the intensity and importance of this relationship. Indeed, it is within the context of this relationship that human sexuality emerges, initially through activity focused on life preservation itself. It is also within this intersubjectivity that the child forms its first self-image, although not yet a gendered image, and that desire is born.[3] The legacy of the preoedipal period is a tendency for sexual fantasy to be charted across the terrain of the woman's body and for the desire of women and men alike to echo a primal childhood wish to decipher and satisfy the mother's desire.

The question of the construction of the feminine Oedipus complex provoked considerable debate among psychoanalysts. Some chose to close Pandora's box and return to the pre-Freudian view that an innate heterosexuality inevitably pushes the girl toward the father.[4] Those theorists who confront the contradiction and seek more complex solutions fall, somewhat schematically, into two divisions. The more orthodox follow the lines of Freud's own analysis, which stressed the role of the castration complex.[5] Whereas in boys the fantasy of castration destroys the Oedipus complex, in girls it makes the formation of a "positive" complex possible. The girl cannot tolerate the "fact" of her castration, which she discovers and slowly comes to accept during the phallic phase. She blames her mother for her condition and depreciates her for being castrated as well. No longer able to believe in the phallic power of her clitoris, she renounces masturbation and, repressing her active desires, turns her passive desires toward her father.

The girl's libido slips into a new position along the line . . . of the equation "penis-child." She gives up her wish for a penis and puts in place of it a wish for a child: and with *that purpose in view* she takes her father as a love object. Her mother becomes an object of jealousy. The girl has turned into a little woman. (*SE* 19:256)

The feminine position, according to Freud, is only really established if the wish for a penis is replaced by the wish for a baby. However, Freud suggested that the wish for a phallus persists in the unconscious in spite of attempts to renounce it. He even contended that penis envy was very possibly impervious to analysis (*SE* 23:250–51).

The other line of explanation, formulated mainly by object-relations theorists, finds the motivation for the girl's turn to the father primarily in the preoedipal mother–child relationship.[6] Here, the fantasy of castration is evoked by an all-powerful mother, and penis envy and the transition to the father as love-object are viewed as being motivated primarily by the girl's wish to free herself from an omnipotent mother. Both sexes fear and suffer a narcissistic wound at the hands of the mother; the boy, however, overcomes this wound through the recognition of the masculinity his phallus represents. The girl, thus, seeks the phallus as a way of individuating from the mother. As Nancy Chodorow explains:

The penis, or phallus, is a symbol of power or omnipotence whether you have one as a sexual organ (as a male) or as a sexual object (as her mother "possesses" her father's). A girl wants it for the powers which it symbolizes and the freedom it promises from her previous sense of dependence, and not because it is inherently and obviously better to be masculine: "Basically, penis envy is the symbolic expression of another desire. Women do not wish to become men, but want to detach themselves from the mother and become complete, autonomous *women.*" A girl's wish to liberate herself from her mother engenders penis envy.[7]

The notion of an omnipotent mother seeking to prevent her child's individuation has a material basis. The changing meaning and structure of the family, and the role of the mother within it, as they have developed in Western capitalist societies over the last two centuries, have resulted in exaggerated centripetal tendencies in the mother–child relationship. There appears, thus, to be a certain plausibility to the suggestion that the girl views the father as a potential liberator.

Ultimately, however, this explanation makes sense only if we abstract away from patriarchal social relations when constructing the analysis; and this is precisely what object-relations theory does. In object-relations theory the triadic structure (father–mother–child) is replaced by the dyadic structure (mother/child) as the elementary relational structure within which gender identity and sexuality are formed. Because of this replacement, patriarchal social relations necessarily lie *outside* the basic unit of analysis and, therefore, play no determining part in the process of forming gender identity and sexuality. They are brought in only after the fact—after these formations have already been accounted for theoretically. Because the content and structure of actual social relations between women and men, and the symbolic representations of these relations, are *left out* of the analytical framework, because the fundamental dilemmas of feminine gender identity and heterosexuality have been defined solely in terms of the girl's preoedipal (read: prepatriarchal) relationship to the mother, the scenario in which the father appears as liberator seems to make sense.[8]

The obvious problem with this, however, is that even if we accept the reasonable proposition that the girl seeks to escape the centripetal and confining nature of her relationship to her mother through the socially acceptable and even socially required route of the turn to the father, the father and the phallus are *not* empty vessels that she can fill with whatever content she pleases—that is, with liberation. They are imbued with social meanings that are, above all, *patriarchal* and that, therefore, militate against liberation by confronting the girl with new and seemingly more permanent forms of imprisonment and dependency. It is precisely these meanings that each girl must come to terms with at the oedipal "moment," and it is these that any adequate theory of the formation of gender identity and sexuality in a patriarchal culture *must* have at the center of its theoretical framework.

Although different in crucial ways, these two tendencies in psychoanalytic theory also share certain common understandings vis-à-vis this particular issue. Both acknowledge that the transition is never really perfectly achieved. Because the feminine Oedipus complex is a secondary formation, women retain more of their original bisexuality. The desire for the mother cannot be totally renounced. Both theories also, however, ultimately stress an ambivalent attitude toward the mother, the legacy of which is a *crippling* ambivalence toward women and toward the self. This is in contrast to a relatively unambivalent coveting of the phallus, either as a means of escape or because the phallus is all there is in a patriarchal culture.

If this latter formulation is essentially complete, the barriers to the successful construction of a feminine Oedipus complex are considerably less formidable than they at first appear. The primary barrier, incestuous desire for the mother, is sufficiently overwhelmed by hostility toward her, on the one hand, and by the desire for the phallus, on the other.

I suggest, however, that this formulation leaves out a crucial element that makes this process far more contradictory. Neither theory seriously considers the possibility of an essential ambivalence toward the phallus itself. However, a close analysis of the fantasies that are integrally intertwined with the Oedipus complex reveals that such ambivalence *must* be the case. Psychoanalytic formulations present the phallus alternatively as signifier of desire, as symbolizing protection, invulnerability, potency, or freedom from an all-engulfing, preoedipal mother. The fantasies of castration and of the Father-as-castrator force us to posit other meanings: violence, destruction, sadism. The primal fantasy of castration depends, on the one hand, upon the equation of femininity, masochism, and annihilation and, on the other, upon the sadistic meaning of the phallus/Father.

These meanings are also clearly expressed in a second fantasy that takes form during the oedipal period and expresses the essential content of patriarchal sexual fantasy. In his analytic work Freud repeatedly discovered a fantasy in the unconscious of his analysands that he termed the "primal scene." The fantasy was the same for men and women; in it, heterosexual union, violence, and degradation were intertwined. J. Laplanche and J.-B. Pontalis define Freud's notion of the "primal scene" as the "scene of sexual intercourse between the parents which the child observes or infers on the basis of certain indications or phantasies. It is generally interpreted by the child as an act of violence on the part of the father."[9] Freud first used the term in his analysis of the Wolf Man, suggesting that sex between the parents is understood by the child as "an aggression by the father in a sado-masochistic relationship," and subsequently he noted: "Among the store of phantasies of all neurotics, and probably of all human beings, this scene is seldom absent" (*SE* 14:269).

Psychoanalytic theory argues that the fantasy of the "primal scene" is in fact a misinterpretation on the child's part, due to the influence of a specific libidinal phase—the anal-sadistic stage. In contrast, I believe it is an accurate perception of the dominant patriarchal sexual fantasy. The fantasy, quite simply, expresses erotically the essential meaning of sexual difference in patriarchal culture. Although the content may vary, the form of "primal scene" fantasies remains constant. Embedded most definitively in pornography, the "scene" is one of dominance and submission, and these are its essential erotic components.[10] Further, gender defines the positions in the "scene." For in its archetypal formulation, the fantasy is heterosexual; it is a "scene" between a man and a woman. Even when those acting out the fantasy are of the same sex, the "scene" depicts the submission and degradation of whoever is in the feminine position. That is to say, ultimately and always, a woman is being degraded. The fantasy may be mild in content, or it may reach to the extreme other end of the continuum to express a sadomasochistic desire that seeks ultimate satisfaction in the total annihilation of the woman—the feminine.

If we view the Oedipus complex from this vantage point, we can see that the complex confronts the child not only with the sexual prohibitions of her or his culture but also with the interconnected meanings of masculinity, femininity, and heterosexuality. Precisely at the "moment" that the girl confronts the demand that she turn from mother to father, the connections between activity, possession of the phallus, sadism, and masculinity, on the one hand, and passivity, castration, masochism, and femininity, on the other, come into sharp focus. After this "moment," sexual fantasy can never again exist ignorant of the implications of gender.

These are the contradictions in barest outline. They are the product of social relations that determine that sexuality will be created in relation to a woman and that sexual fantasy will be molded by and interbound with the social meaning of sexual difference. To understand the ways in which these contradictions are posed to different races and classes of women in different periods, and the ways in which they are worked out, demands more specific levels of analysis. These are, ultimately, historical questions. In the remainder of this essay, I want to explore the way in which the dilemma was framed for Ida Bauer and the way she sought resolution.

DORA'S HYSTERIA

Unfortunately, Freud gives relatively little information about Ida Bauer's early childhood. We know that Ida's first clearly recognizable symptom—nervous asthma—began when she was eight and was accompanied by a character change. Prior to this time she was a "wild-creature," "but after the asthma she became quiet and well behaved" and she began to fall behind her brother in her studies. Freud guessed that Ida had been masturbating until shortly before the nervous asthma appeared. Freud offers only fragmentary information as to the particular influences that resulted in the repression of Ida's masturbatory fantasies and the birth of her hysteria. He suggests, however, that Ida, whose bedroom was close to her parents' at this time, "had overheard her father in his wife's room at night and had heard him . . . breathing hard during coitus."

> I maintained years ago that the dyspnoea and palpitations that occur in hysteria and anxiety-neurosis are only detached fragments of the act of copulation; and in many cases, as in Dora's, I have been able to trace back the symptom of dyspnoea or nervous asthma to the same exciting cause—to the

patient's having overheard sexual intercourse taking place between adults. The sympathetic excitement which may be supposed to have occurred in Dora on such an occasion may very easily have made the child's sexuality veer round and have replaced her inclination to masturbation by an inclination to morbid anxiety. (*SE* 7:79–80; *C* 98)

Yet if this was the precipitating event, it is not clear from Freud's account why Ida would replace "her inclination to masturbation by an inclination to morbid anxiety."

Both changes in character of this kind observed in Ida and the end of masturbation are associated with the final stages of the Oedipus complex in girls. However, although clinical evidence supports the theory that girls cling to the preoedipal period much longer than do boys, until age eight seems a bit too long. Clearly, Ida Bauer had confronted and repressed the oedipal dilemma prior to the appearance of her hysteria. Her hysteria signaled a breakthrough of the repressed oedipal constellation.

The early appearance of Ida's hysterical symptoms is somewhat unusual. The long latency period that separates the oedipal period and puberty can offer a temporary respite from oedipal conflicts. Thus, hysteria and other forms of unconscious conflict often first appear at puberty, when resolution becomes mandatory. However, apparently Ida Bauer was not able to postpone ultimate confrontation with the contradiction that structures postoedipal femininity. At eight, Ida Bauer was trapped in her oedipal struggle and would remain so for life.

We are now confronted with the problem of how Ida Bauer learned the meaning of heterosexuality. The most important source of information clearly was her mother, Käthe Bauer. If name and property were traced through patrilineal descent in Victorian Europe, fantasy was in large part matrilineal.

Quite a few times during the course of the analysis Freud noted that Ida Bauer equated heterosexuality with contamination and self-destruction. Ida knew that her father was syphilitic, and more importantly, she knew how he had become so. She understood that "her father . . . had fallen ill through leading a loose life, and she assumed that he had handed on his bad health to her by heredity." At the point in the analysis when this accusation began to surface, "for several days on end she identified herself with her mother by means of slight symptoms and peculiarities of manner" (*SE* 7:75; *C* 93). Ida remembered a visit she had made to Franzensbad with her mother, who was suffering from abdominal pains and from a discharge. Ida, no doubt correctly, blamed her father for passing on his venereal disease to her mother. One important meaning of Ida's own vaginal discharge, which she periodically fretted over, was an identification with her mother.

Käthe Bauer was clearly obsessed with a fear of contamination: "No one could enter the Bauer apartment without taking off his shoes; on Fridays and other occasions of 'thorough' cleaning, the apartment had to be avoided altogether."[11] Rooms such as the salon, where Philip Bauer kept his cigars, were locked at all times to ensure against contamination. To enter the room Käthe Bauer's permission was necessary, as she had the only key. These obsessional demands were perhaps ways for her to seek control over the destructive phallus. We do not know when these symptoms began; however, the fantasy of heterosexuality as destructive to the woman no doubt began as early for Käthe Bauer as it did for her daughter. She appeared to have been able to sustain a sexual relationship with Philip Bauer for only a few years; by the time he contracted tuberculosis—when Ida was six—they were already estranged.

Käthe Bauer's fantasy, of course, became reality, a fact that was not lost on Ida and that Freud himself acknowledged in passing:

> [Dora] thought her father suffered from veneral disease—for had he not handed it on to her and her mother? She might therefore have imagined to herself that all men suffered from venereal disease. . . . To suffer from venereal disease . . . meant for her to be afflicted with a disgusting discharge. So may we not have here a further motive for the disgust she felt at the moment of the embrace? (*SE* 7:84; *C* 103)

Ida Bauer's fear that all men suffered from venereal disease was not a foolish one. "Sexual diseases" were of epidemic proportions during the late nineteenth and early twentieth centuries, and middle-class women frequently were infected by their husbands. Clearly, one important source of the equation of heterosexuality and contamination for bourgeois women in Victorian Europe was the fact of venereal disease.[12]

Ida Bauer's responses to the two seduction scenes that are the focus of the case, and the hysterical symptoms that were their aftermath, illuminate both her attempted disavowal of and her preoccupation with the sadistic meaning of the phallus and the "primal scene." In the first seduction scene, which took place at Herr K.'s place of business when Ida was fourteen, Herr K.'s kiss aroused in Ida "a violent feeling of disgust." From this response Freud concluded:

> In this scene . . . the behaviour of this child of fourteen was already entirely and completely hysterical. I should without question consider a person hysterical in whom an occasion for sexual excitement elicited feelings that were preponderantly or exclusively unpleasurable; and I should do so whether or no the person were capable of producing symptoms. (*SE* 7:28; *C* 44)

Freud indeed argues here that Ida Bauer was hysterical because she was disgusted by Herr K.'s kiss when she should have felt aroused.[13] Even Freud was somewhat apprehensive about this proposition. He adds quickly: "The elucidation of the mechanism of this *reversal of affect* is one of the most important and at the same time one of the most difficult problems in the psychology of the neurosis. In my judgment, I am still some way from having achieved this end."

Freud also noted that the response displayed a *displacement of sensation*. "Instead of the genital sensation which would certainly have been felt by a healthy girl in such circumstances," Freud writes, "Dora was overcome by the unpleasurable feeling which is proper to the tract of the mucous membrane at the entrance to the alimentary canal—that is by disgust." In addition, "the scene left other consequences in the shape of a sensory hallucination in which she upon occasion could still feel upon the upper part of her body the pressure of Herr K.'s embrace" and a phobia that prevented her from walking past any man and woman engaged in "eager or affectionate conversation." Freud deduced that

> during the man's passionate embrace she felt not merely his kiss upon her lips but also the presence of his erect member against her body. This perception was revolting to her; it was dismissed from her memory, repressed, and replaced by the innocent sensation of pressure upon her thorax. . . . Once

more, therefore, we find a displacement from the lower part of the body to the upper. (*SE* 7:29–30; *C* 45)

Freud's brilliant analysis of Ida Bauer's hysterical symptoms clearly reveals that they were attempts to repudiate the memory of Herr K.'s erection, or, the memory of the phallus. The fact that the sensations are displaced upward to Ida's throat, which is also the focus of her other symptoms, is significant, as we shall see.

Ida Bauer's response to Herr K.'s sexual overtures while she and her father vacationed with the K.'s at the resort lake two years later was equally unambivalent: Ida slapped his face and fled. She also attempted to defend herself from Herr K. while she stayed at the K.'s vacation house by obtaining a key to her room from Frau K.; and she took the first opportunity to leave the K.'s by accompanying her father when he left for home three days later. This last "scene" effectively ended her relationship with Herr and Frau K. and intensified her hysteria to such a degree as to precipitate her analysis with Freud.

In the face of such consistent behavior, why should we follow Freud in his assertion that Ida Bauer's attitude toward Herr K. was not what it appeared to be? That her symptoms revealed *reversal of affect?* Why should we be convinced that her behavior and her desire were at odds?

Freud persistently attempted to demonstrate to Ida that she was in fact in love with Herr K. Freud noted that Ida's coughing attacks lasted from three to six weeks and that this was precisely the duration of Herr K.'s frequent business trips out of town. If Ida's attacks coincided with Herr K.'s absences, then the hidden meaning of the attacks would be a longing for Herr K. Ida allegedly imitated Frau K., who was ill when Herr K. was at home and well when he was away. Ida, Fraud argued, gave her illnesses the opposite meaning. Freud was not able to establish a clear correlation between Ida's attacks and Herr K.'s absences; however, he felt the correlation to be close enough to support his interpretation.

Freud viewed Ida's affection for Herr K.'s children as a "cloak for something else that [Ida] was anxious to hide from herself and from other people," namely, "that she had all these years been in love with Herr K." (*SE* 7:37; *C* 53). While Ida for the most part did not accept this idea, she did tell Freud that other people had told her that she was "simply wild about the man." And finally, under the influence of Freud's persistent prodding, Ida "admitted that she might have been in love with Herr K. . . . but declared that since the scene by the lake it had all been over."

It would be foolish to deny that Ida Bauer formed an attachment to Herr K. or that she was unaware of Herr K.'s growing erotic feelings for her. While it seems very doubtful that "it was possible for Herr K. to send [Ida] flowers every day for a whole year while he was in the neighborhood, to take every opportunity of giving her valuable presents, and to spend all his spare time in her company, without her parents noticing anything in his behavior characteristic of lovemaking" (*SE* 7:35; *C* 51), it seems all but impossible that Ida herself did not notice.

It would be equally foolish, however, to overlook the utilitarian characteristics of this attachment. Ida Bauer's primary task as an adolescent woman was to resolve her sexuality, once and for all, in favor of heterosexuality. Given her hysteria and the *refusal* that lay at its core, her choice of Herr K. was truly ingenious. It allowed her to comply with the demands her family and culture placed upon her while at the same time allowing her to revolt against those demands—and to do so in the name of social propriety and social justice.[14] She could comply with her father's wishes and wear the cloak of femininity by receiving the romantic attentions of Herr K., while knowing full well that this was a doomed affair, for any respectable consummation demanded that Herr K. divorce his wife and marry Ida, and this was highly unlikely, if not impossible, given the strictures of respectable *fin de siècle* Vienna. In this light, Herr K.'s attempts at seduction, which could not have been completely unexpected by Ida, seemed to be ample justification for her rejection of him, as indeed they were. However, this obscured the formidable injustice of patriarchal relations in Victorian Europe, as well as the almost tragic dimensions of her defiance.

Ida Bauer's choice was ingenious in that it served another double function as well, and this function was probably her strongest unconscious motivation. Ida's flirtation with heterosexual romance plummeted her into an erotic triangle with Frau K., while at the same time masking the fact that Frau K. was her primary "object" of desire. Freud, in fact, implicitly recognized this, despite his own formidable resistance. In a series of footnotes, Freud undid his entire analysis by suggesting that behind the "almost limitless series of displacements" that structued Ida Bauer's symptoms and dreams, "it was possible to divine the operation of a single simple factor"—Ida's "deep-rooted homosexual love for Frau K." *(SE 7:105n; 120n; C 126n; 142n.).* He recognized that up until the "scene" by the lake, "the young woman and the scarcely grown girl had lived for years on a footing of closest intimacy. When [Ida] stayed with the K.'s she used to share a bedroom with Frau K., and the husband used to be quartered elsewhere." It was with Frau K., Freud surmised, that Ida had read Mantegazza's *Physiology of Love.* Frau K. had also discussed with Ida the "intimate" problems of her married life, and Ida had often praised Frau K.'s "adorable white body" when she spoke of her to Freud in "accents more appropriate to a lover than to a defeated rival." She also told Freud with pleasure of a time when "evidently through the agency of Frau K. she had been given a present of jewelry [by her father] which was exactly like some that she had seen in Frau K.'s possession and had wished for aloud at the time" (*SE* 7:612; *C* 79).

It seems quite clear that the intimate sexual discussions that occupied so much of Ida and Frau K.'s time alone together had erotic meaning to them both. While the discussions were unquestionably of heterosexual fantasies, these fantasies mediated the sexual relationship between the two women. In essence, the man, be he Philip Bauer or Herr K., who always stood between the two women, in fantasy and in reality, was necessary although superfluous: necessary because he masked the homosexual desires that found some degree of satisfaction in this roundabout way. Necessary also because desire, viewed backward through the prism of the Oedipus complex, is always a triangular affair.

Philip Bauer and Herr K. were crucial to the possibility of the sexual relationship between the two women. Ida was, however, always the weak link in the incestuous triangles that the K.'s and the Bauers formed. When Herr K. demanded that Ida's romantic fantasies succumb to his sexual desire, she blew the whistle, so to speak, on everyone's fantasy—including her own. Frau K. responded by siding with her husband, revealing to him that Ida read Mantegazza and spoke of "forbidden topics." Freud suggested that beneath Ida's accusation of betrayal by her father lay a deeper sense of having been betrayed by Frau K., unconscious because her love was unconscious. And this betrayal echoed an earlier, primal betrayal of being loved not "for her own sake but on account of her father" (*SE* 7:62, *C* 80).[15] In revealing Ida's "preoccupation" with sex to Herr K., Frau K. not only betrayed Ida, but denied the sexual fantasy they had shared together. For it was not Ida alone who was preoccupied with sexual matters and who read Mantegazza, but Ida and Frau K. together. Frau K. did indeed sacrifice their erotic relationship in order to protect herself and to preserve her relationship with Philip Bauer. Frau K.'s actions reiterated with devastating clarity the sexual law of Ida Bauer's culture. Ida's father stood between her and Frau K. as the symbolic Father stands between all women.

Yet, in a sense, Ida Bauer was an outlaw. As Freud noted, Frau K. was the one person whom Ida spared, while she pursued the others with an almost malignant vindictiveness. In sparing Frau K., Ida spared herself. In this way she denied both her love for Frau K. as well as its futility.

DREAMS AND THE DILEMMA

Much of Freud's analysis centered around the interpretation of two dreams that Ida Bauer brought him during the course of the analysis. Both dreams related directly to the "scene" by the lake. In both cases, Freud's interpretation of the latent dream thoughts supported his thesis that Ida Bauer was summoning up her oedipal love for her father to protect her from her love for Herr K. and her desire to surrender to him. A reconsideration of this latent content, even as Freud influenced it, reveals other possibilities. It is not difficult to find in Ida Bauer's two dreams the crystallization of her oedipal struggle: disavowal of the "primal scene" and the breakthrough of repressed lesbian desire.

The first of these two dreams was a recurrent one that Ida remembered first having dreamt three nights in succession after the "scene" by the lake:

> A house was on fire. My father was standing beside my bed and woke me up. I dressed myself quickly. Mother wanted to stop and save her jewel-case; but father said: "I refuse to let myself and my children be burnt for the sake of your jewel-case." We hurried downstairs, and as soon as I was outside I woke up. (*SE* 7:64; *C* 81)

Freud interpreted the dream as a resolution and, more importantly, as a wish. Ida had responded to Herr K.'s proposal on their walk by slapping him in the face and fleeing. Later that day she awoke from a nap in her bedroom to find Herr K. standing beside her. She asked him "sharply" what he wanted, and he replied that he "was not going to be prevented from coming into his bedroom when he wanted." Ida obtained a key to the bedroom from Frau K., but when she wanted to lock herself in to take her afternoon rest, she found that the key had been taken. Naturally she suspected Herr K. The dream occurred for the first time that night. Freud correctly deduced that insofar as the dream represented a resolution, Ida was in that way saying to herself, "I shall have no rest . . . until I am out of this house" (*SE* 7:66–67; *C* 84–85).

There were, however, deeper meanings to the dream, which Freud interpreted through two lines of association. One led back to Ida's childhood memory of her father waking her and Otto up from sleep to take them to the bathroom. This association led Freud to Ida's childhood habit of bed-wetting and his conjecture that it was associated with masturbation. A second line of association led to a dispute between Ida's parents that had occurred when she was fifteen in which her mother rejected a bracelet Philip Bauer had bought for her; she was angry because she had requested that he buy her a particular pair of pearl drop earrings and he had refused. In association with this memory, Ida also remembered that a short time before Herr K. had made her a present of an expensive jewel case. The German word for jewel case, *Schmuckkästchen,* is also a slang expression for the female genitals. Thus Freud deduced that in Ida's dream jewel case represented her vagina, her virginity, and sexual intercourse. Using these associations, he made the following analysis of the main dream wish:

> You said to yourself: "This man is persecuting me; he wants to force his way into my room. My 'jewel-case' is in danger, and if anything happens it will be father's fault." For that reason in the dream you chose a situation which expresses the opposite—a danger from which your father is saving you. In this part of the dream everything is turned into its opposite; you will soon discover why. As you say, the mystery turns upon your mother. You ask how she comes into the dream? She is, as you know, your former rival in your father's affections. In the incident of the bracelet you would have been glad to accept what your mother had rejected. Now let us just put "give" instead of "accept" and "withhold" instead of "reject." Then it means that you were ready to give your father what your mother withheld from him. Now bring your mind back to the jewel-case which Herr K. gave you. You have there the starting-point for a parallel line of thoughts, in which Herr K. is to be put in place of your father just as he was in the manner of standing beside your bed. He gave you a jewel-case; so you are ready to give Herr K. what his wife withholds from him. That is the thought which has made it necessary for every one of its elements to be turned into its opposite.

And what is the upshot of this analysis? Freud concluded to Ida:

> You are summoning up your old love for your father in order to protect yourself aginst your love for Herr K. But what do all these efforts show? Not only that you are afraid of Herr K., but that you are still more afraid of the temptation you feel to yield to him. In short these efforts prove once more how deeply you loved him. (*SE* 7:69–70; *C* 87–88)

Freud's analysis of the hidden dream wish did not strike a responsive chord in Ida Bauer; Freud conceded that Ida "would not follow me in this part of the interpretation." He held to it nonetheless.

One can never, of course, disprove a dream interpretation, especially three-quarters of a century after the fact. However, I also find that I cannot follow Freud. The main problem lies with the role of the mother in the dream. "*Mother wanted to stop and save her jewel-case, but father said: 'I refuse to let myself and my children be burnt for the sake of your jewel-case.'*" Freud suggested that in one important sense Frau K. is really the mother in the dream, and on one level the suggestion makes sense. No doubt Ida wished that her father would end his barter with Herr K. by saying similar words to Frau K. But the fact that the mother is trying to save her jewel case in the dream needs further explanation. If we consider this phrase in light of the suggestion that for Käthe Bauer, as for Ida, heterosexuality equaled contamination and destruction, the dream takes on another meaning. The mother's attempt to save her "jewel case" can have no other meaning—given this shared fantasy—than an attempt to escape heterosexuality and annihilation. Beneath Ida's wish that her father save her jewel-case lies the recognition that he, in fact, demands its destruction, as he demands the destruction of her mother's. The assocation leading back to Ida's bed-wetting is relevant. It is possible that the memory of Philip Bauer waking Ida to take her to the bathroom may have hidden another memory of her being awakened by her parents' "lovemaking." Freud does argue that this was the trauma that initiated Ida's hysteria. Certainly Ida Bauer understood only too well the meaning such sexual encounters had for Käthe Bauer, and it was a meaning she appropriated as her own. This is underscored by the association to the argument between Käthe and Philip Bauer over his gift of jewelry. Insofar as this scene was a metaphor for sex, as Freud argues, the most significant aspect of the scene is Käthe Bauer's rejection of her husband's "gift."

The association leading back to Ida's bed-wetting and masturbation is also important because it refers to the last period in which Ida expresssed sexuality in an active, conscious way. In the dream, Ida's father is presented as saving her from fire, from sexuality, as he did when he awoke her and her brother as children. But, in fact, her father, insofar as he represented the symbolic Father, forced Ida to relinquish her preoedipal sexuality and to renounce its object. At the deepest level of meaning in the dream, Ida's father is represented as the enforcer of the (hetero)sexual laws and fantasies of Ida Bauer's culture.

A few sessions before Ida terminated the analysis, she brought Freud her second dream.

I was walking about in a town which I did not know. I saw streets and squares which were strange to me. Then I came into a house where I lived, went to my room, and found a letter from Mother lying there. She wrote saying that as I had left home without my parents' knowledge she had not wished to write to me to say that Father was ill. "Now he is dead, and if you like you can come." I then went to the station and asked about a hundred times: "Where is the station?" I always got the answer: "Five minutes." I then saw a thick wood before me which I went into, and there I asked a man whom I met. He said to me: "Two and a half hours more." He offered to accompany me. But I refused and went alone. I saw the station in front of me and could not reach it. At the same time I had the usual feeling of anxiety that one has in dreams when one cannot move forward. Then I was at home. I must have been travelling in the meantime, but I know nothing about that. I walked into the porter's lodge, and inquired for our flat. The maidservant opened the door to me and replied that Mother and the others were already at the cemetery. I saw myself particularly distinctly going up the stairs. After she answered I went to my room, but not the least sadly, and began reading a big book that lay on my writing table. (*SE* 7:94; *C* 114).

Among Ida's associations, the most important are these:

First, wandering in a strange town related to her memory of a brief visit to Dresden. "On that occasion she had been a stranger and had wandered about, not failing, of course, to visit the famous picture gallery. [A] cousin of hers . . . had wanted to act as a guide and take her round the gallery. *But she declined and went alone,* and stopped in front of the pictures that appealed to her. She remained *two hours* in front of the Sistine Madonna, rapt in silent admiration. When I asked her what had pleased her so much about the picture she could find no clear answer to make. At last she said, 'The Madonna.' " (*SE* 7:96; *C* 116).

Second, the letter in the dream recalled both Ida's own suicide note and the letter she had received from Frau K. inviting her to the resort lake. In that letter Frau K. had placed a question mark in the middle of a sentence after the phrase, "if you would like to come," just as it appeared in her amended version of the dream.

Third, the thick wood in the dream was like the wood by the shore of the lake where Herr K. made his proposal. Ida had also seen the very same wood the day before in a picture at the Secessionist exhibition. In the background of the picture, however, there had been nymphs.

Freud suggested that two fantasies structured the dream. The first was a fantasy of revenge against Ida's father, represented by his death in the dream. Freud argued that the associations relating to the thick wood in the dream suggested a second fantasy of defloration—"the phantasy of a man seeking to force an entrance into the female genitals." In German the same word, *nymphae,* represents both "nymphs," which were in the background of one of the paintings at the Secessionist exhibition, and *Nymphae,* the technical term for labia minora. Thus at the core of this dream is the "primal scene"—but a particular version appropriate to Ida Bauer's circumstances.

Freud concluded that Ida could only have gotten the technical term *Nymphae* from reading anatomical textbooks or from an encyclopedia—the big book she goes to her room in order to read in the dream—and connected the two fantasies, revenge and defloration, to the meaning of this reading act:

> Parents are very much in the way while reading of this kind is going on. But this uncomfortable situation had been radically improved, thanks to the dream's power of fulfilling wishes. Dora's father was dead, and the others had already gone to the cemetery. She might calmly read whatever she chose. Did not this mean that one of her motives for revenge was a revolt against her parents' [father's] constraint? If her father was dead she could read or love as she pleased. (*SE* 7:100; *C* 121)

Ida did not wish just to read about the "primal scene," however; she also wished to experience it. Freud suggested that an important key to the meaning of the dream is the association to the Sistine Madonna. The Madonna, Freud argued, was obviously Ida herself. The identification revealed Ida's concern with her virginity; it also, however, represented her wish for a child. Ida had won Herr K.'s affection by the motherliness she had shown toward his children, and "she had had a child though she was still a girl" *(SE* 9:104*n; C* 125*n.).* This last reference is to Ida's false appendicitis attack, which occurred shortly after her aunt's death and nine months after the "scene" by the lake and left Ida with a limp that periodically returned. Freud interpreted the attack as a fantasy of childbirth. Ida, he argued, regretted not having surrendered to Herr K. at the lake and in her unconscious fantasy life acted as though she had. The limp symbolized her "false step." Once again Freud concluded to Ida: "So you see that your love for Herr K. did not come to an end with the scene, but that (as I maintained) it has persisted down to the present day—though it is true that you are unconscious of it" (*SE* 7:104; *C* 125).

Writing of hysteria thirty years later, Freud made a very different argument:

> It is not hard to show that another regression to an earlier level occurs in hysteria. . . . The sexuality of female children is dominated and directed by a masculine organ (the clitoris) and often behaves like the sexuality of boys. This masculine sexuality has to be got rid of by a last wave of development at puberty, and the vagina . . . has to be raised into the dominant erotogenic zone. Now it is very common in hysterical neurosis for this repressed masculine sexuality to be reactivated and then for the defensive struggle on the part of the ego-syntonic instincts to be directed against it. (*SE* 12:325–26)

I do not want to discuss Freud's notion that the clitoris is a "masculine" organ and that the sexuality attached to it is "masculine." Freud was, of course, well aware that we cannot really talk of masculinity and femininity as we know it as adults until after the Oedipus complex. What Freud calls "masculine sexuality" is really preoedipal sexuality in which the "primal scene" and the meaning of the difference between the sexes are not yet fully comprehended and in which the mother or mother surrogate is the primary object of desire. During the later stages of this period, during the phallic phase, both girls and boys direct a genital sexuality with passive and active aims toward their mother, whose physical ministrations make her the first seducer. However, the little girl wants not only to be seduced by the mother but also to seduce her in turn.

> Intense *active* wishful impulses directed towards the mother also arise during the phallic phase. The sexual activity of this period culminates in clitoridal masturbation. This is probably accompanied by ideas of the mother, but whether

the child attached a sexual aim to the idea, and what the aim is, I have not been able to discover from my observations. It is only when all her interests have received fresh impetus through the arrival of a baby brother or sister that we can clearly recognize such an aim. The little girl wants to believe that she has given her mother the new baby, just as the boy wants to. (*SE* 21:239)

By Freud's own admission, the deepest level of meaning of hysterical symptoms is not a thwarted desire for the father, but a breakthrough of the prohibited desire for the mother. If we consider the dream from this point of view, it is immediately obvious that the dream is a crystallization of Ida Bauer's oedipal struggle. On one level, the dream is a clear symbolization and rejection of the "primal scene" and the feminine position Ida must assume in it. It is clear, however, that she does not assume this position in the dream. As Freud pointed out, "What was most evident was that in the first part of the dream she was identifying herself with a young man . . . wandering about in a strange place . . . striving to reach a goal. . . . It would have been appropriate for the goal to have been the possession of a woman" (*SE* 7:96–97; *C* 116–17). Freud argued that in this part of the dream Ida is identifying with a young suitor of hers who had sent her a picture that forms the imagery of the strange town in which Ida is wandering in the beginning of the dream. Insofar as the underlying fantasy is one of defloration, Freud is suggesting that, to the extent that Ida takes a place in the "scene," she takes the place of the man.

The letter from Ida's mother telling her "now he [Ida's father] is dead, and if you like? you can come," was directly associated with Frau K.'s letter inviting Ida to vacation with her and Herr K. in the Alps. Certainly the obvious underlying thought was that if her father disappeared she would have Frau K. to herself. Insofar as Frau K.'s betrayal of Ida, which was precipitated by Herr K.'s proposal, replayed an earlier oedipal scenario, Ida's wish that her father die was not only a fantasy of revenge, as Freud suggested, but also a wish to create another sort of reality. This is one of the meanings of the Sistine Madonna in Ida's dream. For the image of the Madonna and Child is a preoedipal phantasy that suggests oral sexuality. This image, as well as the location of Ida Bauer's hysterical symptoms—chronic cough, gastric pains, mild anorexia—indicate that the conflict, which was framed in terms of genital sexuality, was transposed to and played out on the oral terrain. Ida's fantasy of the lovemaking of Frau K. and her father, which Freud interpreted as taking the form of fellatio, also suggests this. This transposition was an attempt to deny the phallus and the Father by constructing a mythical world where the mother/child dyad could exist undisturbed by the implications of sexual difference.

The fantasy of the Madonna denies the phallus in another way as well. Freud pointed out that the fantasy is one of a *virgin* mother. We could put the point differently, however, and call it a fantasy of *immaculate conception,* that is, a conception in which the phallus and the "primal scene" play no role.[16] Is this not the solution to Ida Bauer's dilemma? The Madonna found her way into Ida Bauer's dream precisely because she represented the negation of the "primal scene"—the negation of masculinity and femininity.

Ida's second dream reveals that her attempts to escape the implications of femininity oscillated between attempted retreats to oral sexuality and hysterical identifications with masculinity (identification with her own suitor). Neither provided the possibility of a real resolution, however. These efforts to escape were contrasted with efforts to comply—that is, with hysterical identifications with femininity, revealed not only in Ida's identification with her mother but also in her false appendicitis attack, occurring shortly after the death of Ida's favorite aunt, and nine months after Herr K.'s proposal at the lake.[17] Freud interpreted the attack as a childbirth fantasy representing Ida's wish that she had surrendered to Herr K., and the limp, which periodically appeared after the attack, as a metaphor for the impropriety of her desire, her "false step." That Ida's hysterical attack occurred nine months after Herr K.'s proposal does indeed indicate that one crucial meaning was a fantasy of childbirth. The question is whether this fantasy necessarily implies that Ida Bauer had in fact regretted her response to Herr K.'s proposal.

At the beginning of a session that Freud planned to devote to the interpretation of Ida's second dream, she announced that she was terminating the analysis. She had made the decision two weeks earlier but had said nothing to Freud. Freud suggested that "that sounds just like a maidservant or governess—a fortnight's warning." The suggestion proved illuminating. Ida remembered that during her stay at the lake a governess in service with the K.'s had given notice to Herr K., who had seduced her, "saying that he got nothing from his wife" (*SE* 7:106; *C* 127), the very same words he used later to proposition Ida. When Herr K. quickly tired of the governess, she told her parents, who at first demanded that she return home. But she waited a while before giving notice, hoping that Herr K.'s attitude toward her would change, and they disowned her.

Freud concluded, correctly I think, that much of Ida's conduct after the "scene" by the lake, and an important element in her fantasies, represented an identification with this particular servant as well as with servant women in general. Ida told her parents about Herr K.'s proposal just as the servant had written to her parents; and Ida waited two weeks before telling them, just as the governess had waited before giving Herr K. notice. In the dream, the letter inviting Ida home was the counterpart to the letter to the governess from her parents forbidding her to come home. Ida's false appendicitis attack nine months after the "scene" by the lake was also an identification with this female servant. The identification suggests that in Ida's unconscious, servitude and femininity formed a symbolic equation.

This symbolism was not idiosyncratic and had a material basis in historical circumstances. Freud recognized in a letter to Wilhelm Fliess in 1897 that his female analysands often identified in this way:

> An immense load of guilt, with self-reproaches (for theft, abortions, etc.) is made possible for the woman by identification with these people of low morals, who are so often remembered by her as worthless women connected sexually with her father or brother. And, as a result of the sublimation of these girls in phantasies, most improbable charges against other people are made in these phantasies. Fear of prostitution (i.e., of becoming a prostitute), fear of being in the street alone, fear of a man hidden under the bed, etc., also point in the direction of servant-girls. There is a tragic justice in the fact that the action of the head of the family in stooping to a servant girl is atoned for by his daughter's self-abasement. (*SE* 1:248–49)

The passage reveals, as does Ida Bauer's identification, that femininity was linked with service specifically with regard to sexuality. That is, what lies at the heart of these identifications is a particular fantasy of heterosexuality as service due men, and one explicitly based on submission and degradation.

Leonore Davidoff has suggested that the striking tendency in Victorian bourgeois ideology to an exaggerated dual vision of women had a material basis not only in the larger class structure but also in the division of labor within the Victorian bourgeois family itself. During the latter half of the nineteenth century, domestic service became an almost exclusively female profession. Increasingly, domestic servants, who were predominantly young and unmarried, took over tasks involving manual labor and the routine aspects of child care from bourgeois wives:

> It was the nurse or maid who fed, nappied, washed, dressed, potted, put to bed, and directly disciplined the infant and small child. Within the nursery domain she had total power over her charges; yet middle-class children learned very quickly that she was their inferior and that they were both . . . subject to higher authority. It was very often these girls and women who first awakened sexual as well as other feelings in the child.[18]

Davidoff is fundamentally concerned with the impact this actual split had on bourgeois male sexuality and psychology. This included the tendency not only to create the polar oppositions of desexualized Madonna and erotic Magdalen but also to search for a degraded erotic object, that is, fantasy of sexuality as debasement.

If we consider what implications such splitting might have for bourgeois women, we can perceive at once the paradox. Bourgeois women enjoyed the same prerogatives of command and dominance that being members of the ruling class afforded their husbands, fathers, and brothers. They found self-affirmation in the deference showed them by servants who

> stood when spoken to and kept their eyes cast down, they moved out of a room backwards, curtsied to their betters, and were generally expected to efface themselves, doing their work and moving about the house so as not to be visible or audible to their employers. In an extreme case they were made to turn their faces to the wall when the employer passed by.[19]

But gender and class, femininity and service, were at the same time conflated—insofar as the question posed was sexuality. Bourgeois sexual fantasy did not distinguish between classes of women. In this historical circumstance, class and gender intertwined to magnify dramatically the content of the "primal scene."[20]

Freud argued that, in her identification with the K.'s governess, Ida Bauer revealed her desire to submit to Herr K. Yet the logic of Ida's personal history suggests that Ida's identification stemmed not from desire but from the unconscious belief that femininity, bondage, and debasement were synonymous. In her hysterical identification with the K.'s governess, Ida Bauer acted out the drama of femininity. She impersonated the young servant woman, whom she imagined had been seduced by her desire for Herr K., and in exchange for satisfaction had suffered a woman's fate. If her identification symbolized a wish, perhaps she wished she could reconstitute her desire as patriarchy demanded, so that she might reclaim sexuality. But Ida Bauer's frigidity marked the depth of her protest.

In Freud's analysis, the reason for Ida Bauer's protest is repressed. However, in his choice of a pseudonym for Ida Bauer, Freud revealed his own unconscious understanding of one contradiction that aided in the birth of her hysteria. In *The Psychopathology of Everyday Life,* Freud disclosed that when he searched for a name for Ida Bauer, "Dora was the only name to occur" (*SE* 6:241). Dora was the name of a servant in the Freud family who had been his sister's nursemaid. She had been forced to give up her own name, Rosa, as it was also his sister's name. Through his choice, or lack of choice, Freud revealed his recognition that in his mind, as in Ida Bauer's, servitude was a metaphor for femininity. At the very same moment, however, Freud also confessed his wish that like Rosa, the servant woman who gave up even her name, Ida Bauer make her peace with servitude. To escape a feminine fate is the prerogative of the son, not the daughter.

Each time I reread Freud's study, I am struck, as others have been, by one statement Freud makes in the postscript. After tying up every loose end in the analysis, after skillfully introjecting the same meaning into Ida Bauer's every symptom, every action, every unconscious and conscious thought, Freud acknowledges, "I do not know what kind of help she wanted from me." Because of the meaning Freud gave to Ida Bauer's desire, she remained a mystery to him.

Writing of hysteria in our own time, a disciple of Freud voices a similar sentiment: "Hysteria, he writes, " still poses similar difficulties to those of the past, though they are perhaps more sophisticated." "Hysteria still provides the analyst with the illusion of power which the patient takes away after having tempted him to believe he possessed it. Hysteria's subtle intrigue obliges one to overcome a prejudice, to solve a mystery, but, in the end, this is perhaps the mystery of femininity."[21] But is the mystery really so insoluble, or is it perhaps that its solution would demand the shattering of a precious fantasy?

Precious to some, painful to others.

Notes

1. See for example, Erik Erikson's essay in this book, as well as articles by Langs, Laplanche, Lewin, Muslin and Gill, and Slipp listed in the Bibliography.

2. See Juliet Mitchell, *Psychoanalysis and Feminism* (New York: Pantheon, 1974). Mitchell's important contribution to feminist theory was her insight that classical psychoanalysis, which has as one objective of study the formation of gender identity and sexuality in patriarchal culture, is a useful tool for feminism. The critical task is to separate those aspects of the theory that are ideological from those that are insightful and useful—if incomplete. Steven Marcus began the feminist critique of this case history with his perceptive article, "Freud and Dora: Story, History, Case History," in *Representations* (New York: Random House, 1976). This essay has influenced my reading of the case considerably. Recent feminist rereadings of the case include Hélène Cixous, *Portrait de Dora*, and articles by Jacqueline Rose (essay 6 in this book), Hannah S. Decker, ("Freud and Dora"), and Temma Kaplan (see Bibliography for all three).

3. See Jean Laplanche's *Life and Death in Psychoanalysis*, Jeffrey Mehlman, tr. (Baltimore: Johns Hopkins University Press, 1976). Freud's main essays on female sexuality and femininity are "Some Psychical Consequences of the Anatomical Distinction between the Sexes," "Female Sexuality," and "Femininity," all in *SE* 19 and 21. Also see Juliet Mitchell, "On Freud and the Distinction between the Sexes," in *Women and Analysis*, Jean Strouse, ed. (New York: Dell, 1974), p. 46.

4. See, for example, Karen Horney, *Feminine Psychology*, Harold Kelman, ed. (New York: Norton, 1967); and Ernest Jones, *Papers on Psychoanalysis* (Baltimore: Williams and Wilkins, 1950).

5. This line of argument is presented in Mitchell, *Psychoanalysis and Feminism*, and by Gayle Rubin, "The Traffic in Women: Notes on the 'Political Economy' of Sex,"

in *Toward an Anthropology of Women*, Rayna R. Reiter, ed. (New York: Monthly Review Press, 1975).

6. This line of argument has found favor with psychoanalytically oriented North American feminist theorists. It is cogently presented by Nancy Chodorow, *The Reproduction of Mothering: Psychoanalysis and the Sociology of Gender* (Berkeley: University of California Press, 1978); and by Dorothy Dinnerstein, *The Mermaid and the Minotaur: Sexual Arrangements and Human Malaise* (New York: Harper Colophon Books, 1977); also by Jane Flax, "The Conflict Between Nurturance and Autonomy in Mother–Daughter Relationships and Within Feminism," *Feminist Studies* (June 1978), 4(2):171–189. The argument is made in popular form by Nancy Friday, *My Mother/My Self* (New York: Delacorte Press, 1977).

For prominent examples of object-relations theory, see Melanie Klein, *Contributions to Psycho-Analysis, 1921–1945* (London: Hogarth Press, 1948); W. R. D. Fairbairn, *An Object-Relations Theory of the Personality* (New York: Basic Books, 1952); Margaret Mahler, *On Human Symbiosis and the Vicissitudes of Individuation*, Vol. 1, *Infantile Psychosis* (New York: International Universities Press, 1968); D. W. Winnicott, *Playing and Reality* (New York: Basic Books, 1971); and Michael Balint, ed., *Primary Love and Psycho-Analytic Technique* (New York: Liveright, 1965).

7. Chodorow, *Reproduction of Mothering*, p. 123. Chodorow is citing Janine Chasseguet-Smirgel, "Feminine Guilt and the Oedipus Complex," in *Female Sexuality*, J. Chasseguet-Smirgel, ed. (Ann Arbor: University of Michigan Press, 1970), p. 118.

8. This "slippage" leads these theories, and the feminists who use them, to focus primarily on mother–daughter and mother–son ambivalence. At the same time, this focus results in a tendency to explain crucial aspects of the social whole as being fundamentally determined by the dynamics of this single relationship. Thus Chodorow and Dinnerstein locate the origins and reproduction of misogyny in the mother–child relationship.

9. J. Laplanche and J. B. Pontalis, *The Language of Psychoanalysis*, Donald Nicholson-Smith, tr. (New York: Norton, 1973), p. 335. The subsequent quote is from this same page.

10. See Steven Marcus' classic study of sexuality and pornography in nineteenth-century England, *The Other Victorians* (New York: Basic Books, 1964).

11. See Arnold Rogow, "A Further Footnote to Freud's 'Fragment of an Analysis of a Case of Hysteria'," *Journal of the American Psychoanalytic Association* 26(1978), p. 343.

12. Unfortunately, statistics on the frequency of venereal diseases during this period are unreliable and fragmentary. In the early 1900s, Christabel Pankhurst suggested in a pamphlet reprinted from *The Suffragette* that from 75 to 80 percent of British men were infected with gonorrhea, and a considerable percentage were infected with syphilis. The estimate is no doubt inflated for polemical purposes. See J. A. Banks and Olive Banks, *Feminism and Family Planning in Victorian England* (Liverpool: Liverpool University Press, 1964), p. 112. Abraham Flexner's study of prostitution in

Europe at the turn of the century found venereal disease to be most prevalent in the large European cities of Paris, Vienna, and Berlin, where prostitution was under government regulation. Although he cites no statistics for Vienna, he quotes a study which calculated that of the clerks and merchants in Berlin between 18 and 28 years of age, 45 percent had had syphilis and 100 percent had had gonorrhea. Another study estimated that, in Germany, one man in every five contracted syphilis and that gonorrhea averaged more than one attack per man. See Abraham Flexner, *Prostitution in Europe* (New York: Century, 1914), p. 367.

13. Many analysts who have commented on this part of Freud's analysis have argued that Freud's main deficiency was his inability to place Ida Bauer developmentally. Marcus notes, "At one moment in the passage [Freud] calls her a 'girl,' at another a 'child'—but in point of fact he treats her throughout as if this fourteen-, sixteen-, and eighteen-year-old adolescent had the capabilities for sexual response of a grown woman." Another reviewer has suggested that Freud's libidinous countertransferences prevented him from recognizing the absurdity of his expectations that Ida, at fourteen, respond sexually to Herr K. as would a "mature woman." See Hyman Muslin and Merton Gill, "Transference in the Dora Case," *Journal of the American Psychoanalytic Association* 26 (1978), p. 324.

Although objections along this line have validity, particularly with regard to this scene, they prove problematic in light of Ida Bauer's prior and subsequent development. At what age, we may ask, should Ida the "girl" have become Ida the "mature woman," sexually speaking? If Ida Bauer had been repulsed at Herr K.'s embrace when twenty-one, would she then, by this theory, have been hysterical? If Ida's symptoms were the result of her inability to deal with the unspoken pressure that her father exerted to make her submit to Herr K., her hysteria might have begun when she first understood the nature of the barter. It would have abated once she had asserted her will in the matter. But, in fact, Ida's symptoms began when she was eight and continued to plague her throughout her life. The point is that we must interpret the meaning of Ida Bauer's response to this particular scene within the context of her entire history of hysteria.

14. Recent feminist discussions of hysteria stress its element of compliance; see, for example, Decker, "Freud and Dora," pp. 453–454. Hysteria as simple compliance is argued in Luce Irigaray, *Speculum de l'autre femme* (Paris: Minuit, 1974). For an excellent critique of Irigaray's position, see Monique Plaza, " 'Phallomorphic' Power and the Psychology of 'Woman,' " *Feminist Issues* (Summer 1980), no. 1.

15. This betrayal by Frau K. duplicated at least one prior betrayal by a woman. Ida had been on intimate terms with her governess, who "used to read every book on sexual life and similar subjects, and talked to the girl about them," while demanding secrecy from Ida about these goings-on. When Ida discovered that the governess was secretly in love with her father and, she supposed, indifferent to her, Ida had her fired. Freud noted that Ida's own behavior toward Frau and Herr K.'s two children owed something to an identification with this governess. She was the

first of two servant women with whom Ida would make such an identification. See *SE* 7:36, 60; *C* 52, 78.

16. Juliet Mitchell, reviewing Karl Abraham's work on femininity, makes a passing reference to fantasies of immaculate conception as representing an unconscious attempt to deny the importance of the phallus. Such disavowal reveals, of course, a protest against the social meaning of sexual difference. See Mitchell, *Psychoanalysis and Feminism*, p. 124. [The actual dogma of the "immaculate conception" has nothing to do with a phallus or anyone being born of a virgin. It refers to the birth of Mary herself and means that she was born without the curse of original sin. Most people are confused about this and in popular parlance it is associated with virgin birth—Eds.]

17. Unfortunately, our ability to interpret the attack at all its levels of meaning is hindered by the fact that Freud was unable to unearth the line of association that must have existed linking Ida's attack and her aunt's death. This aunt, who Freud informs us in the beginning of the case has been the model upon which Ida patterned her hysteria, is conspicuous by her absence in Ida's unconscious. Yet she must have had important meaning to Ida if Ida copied her unconscious metaphors so closely. Freud noted that part of the material for Ida's second dream was derived directly from Ida's memory of her aunt's death; yet the meaning of this memory is not evident.

18. Leonore Davidoff, "Class and Gender in Victorian England: The Diaries of Arthur J. Munby and Hannah Cullwick," *Feminist Studies* (Spring 1979), 5(1):94.

19. Davidoff, p. 97.

20. Recently, the stereotype of the sexually frigid bourgeois woman has been challenged by F. Barry Smith, "Sexuality in Britain, 1880–1900: Some Suggested Revisions," in *The Widening Sphere: Changing Roles of Victorian Women*, Martha Vicinus, ed. (Bloomington: University of Indiana Press, 1977); and Carl Degler, "What Ought to Be and What Was: Women's Sexuality in the Nineteenth Century," *American Historical Review* (December 1974), 79:1469–1490. Such critical questionings of traditional stereotypes are crucial. However, it will be essential, I think, to bring to the historical evidence some theory of the genesis and nature of human sexuality in general, and of female sexuality in particular. If we discover that hysteria did indeed occur among this class of women often enough to warrant considering it a historically significant phenomenon, then we will have to explore the conjecture that the historical circumstances in which Victorian bourgeois women found themselves tended to exacerbate problems inherent in the development of female sexuality. Hysteria would represent an extreme response.

21. René Major, "Revolution of Hysteria," *International Journal of Psychoanalysis* (1974), 55:391.

8. Representation of Patriarchy: Sexuality and Epistemology in Freud's Dora

TORIL MOI

Over the past few years Freud's account of his treatment of the eighteen-year-old Dora has provoked many feminists to take up their pen, in anger or fascination. Dora had for some time suffered from various hysterical symptoms (nervous cough, loss of voice, migraine, depression, and what Freud calls "hysterical unsociability" and "*taedium vitae*"), but it was not until the autumn of 1900, when her parents found a suicide note from her, that Dora's father sent her to Freud for treatment. Freud's case history reveals much about the situation of a young woman from the Viennese bourgeoisie at the turn of the century. Dora's psychological problems can easily be linked to her social background. She has very little, if any, scope for independent activity, is strictly guarded by her family, and feels under considerable pressure

This essay was first published in *Feminist Review* (1981), 9:60–73. The main sources were oral: it would never have been written were it not for the invaluable insight I gained both from Neil Hertz's seminars on "Freud and Literature" at Cornell University in the fall semester of 1980, and from the exciting and extremely inspiring discussions in the Women's Group on Psychoanalysis at Cornell that same autumn.

from her father. She believes (and Freud agrees) that she is being used as a pawn in a game between her father and Herr K., the husband of her father's mistress. The father wants to exchange Dora for Frau K. ("If I get your wife, you get my daughter"), so as to be able to carry on his affair with Frau K. undisturbed. Dora claims that her father only sent her to psychiatric treatment because he hoped that she would be "cured" into giving up her opposition to her father's affair with Frau K., accept her role as a victim of the male power game, and take Herr K. as her lover.

Freud, then, becomes the person who is to help Dora handle this difficult situation. But Freud himself is the first to admit that his treatment of Dora was a failure. Freud has his own explanations of this failure, but these are not wholly convincing. Feminists have been quick to point out that the reasons for Freud's failure are clearly sexist: Freud is authoritarian, a willing participant in the male power game conducted between Dora's father and Herr K., and at no time turns to consider Dora's own experience of the events. That Freud's analysis fails because of its inherent sexism is the common feminist conclusion.

But *Dora* is a complex text, and feminists have stressed quite different points in their reading of it. Hélène Cixous and Catherine Clément discuss the political potential of hysteria in their book *La jeune née* and agree that Dora's hysteria developed as a form of protest, a silent revolt against male power.[1] They differ, however, as I shall show later, in their evaluation of the importance of hysteria as a political weapon. Cixous and Clément do not discuss in any detail the interaction between Freud and Dora, but Hélène Cixous returned to this theme in 1976, when she published her play *Portrait de Dora.*[2] Here Dora's story is represented in dreamlike sequences from Dora's own viewpoint. Cixous plays skillfully with Freud's text: she quotes, distorts, and displaces the "father text" with great formal mastery. This technique enables her to create new interpretations of Dora's symptoms in a playful exposure of Freud's limitations.

Jacqueline Rose's article, "Dora: Fragment of an Analysis" (see essay 6 in this book), differs considerably from these two French texts. Rose sees *Dora* as a text that focuses with particular acuteness on the problem of the representation of femininity and discusses several modern

French psychoanalytical theories of femininity (particularly Michèle Montrelay and Luce Irigaray in relation to Lacan). She concludes by rejecting that simplistic reading of *Dora* which would see Dora the woman opposed to and oppressed by Freud the man. According to Rose, *Dora* reveals how Freud's concept of the feminine was incomplete and contradictory, thus delineating a major problem in psychoanalytical theory: its inability to account for the feminine. A valuable contribution to a feminist reading of psychoanalysis, Rose's essay is nevertheless silent on its political consequences.

The same is true of Suzanne Gearhart's "The Scene of Psychoanalysis: The Unanswered Questions of Dora" (see essay 5). Gearhart reads *Dora* principally through Lacan's and Irigaray's discussions of Dora's case, arguing that the central problem in the text is "the symbolic status of the father." According to Gearhart, *Dora* must be seen as Freud's "interrogation of the principle of paternity"; it is in the correct understanding of the text's handling of this problem that we will find the key to the ultimate explanation of Dora's illness and also the basis of the identity of Freud and his work. Gearhart's highly sophisticated reading of *Dora* shows that the status of the father in *Dora* is problematical, and the father himself made marginal, because Freud wants to avoid the central insight that the (Lacanian) Imaginary and Symbolic realms are fundamentally complicit. Theoretically valuable though this essay is, it fails to indicate the consequences of its reading of *Dora* for a feminist approach to psychoanalysis.

Maria Ramas' long study of Dora, "Freud's Dora, Dora's Hysteria" (see essay 7), is the most accessible article on Dora to date. Whereas Rose and Gearhart use a sophisticated theoretical vocabulary, Ramas writes in a lucid, low-key style. But her "theoretical" inquiry advances little beyond a scrupulous, somewhat tedious resumé of Freud's text. Ramas argues that "Ida's problem [Ramas uses Dora's real name, Ida Bauer, throughout her text] was her unconscious belief that "femininity, bondage, and debasement were synonymous." Since Freud unconsciously shared this belief, she claims, he could only reinforce Dora's problems rather than free her from them.

This, at least, is a traditional feminist reading: it implies that Dora could escape her hysteria only through feminist consciousness-raising—that if she could stop equating femininity with bondage she would be liberated. But it is also a sadly partial and superficial account, failing to encompass many controversial areas of Freud's text. Despite one brief reference to Jacqueline Rose's article, Ramas seems to find the status of the term *femininity* in the text quite unproblematical; she unquestioningly accepts Freud's automatic reduction of oral sex to fellatio (a point I shall return to later) and does not even notice many of Freud's more eccentric concerns in the case study. Qualifying her own essay as pure "feminist polemics," Ramas suggests that further study of *Dora* would lead beyond feminism: "If this were Freud's story, we would have to go beyond feminist polemics and search for the sources of the negative countertransference—the unanalyzed part of Freud—that brought the analysis to an abrupt end."[3]

I believe that it is precisely through an exploration of the "unanalyzed part of Freud" that we may uncover the relations between sexual politics and psychoanalytical theory in *Dora*, and therefore also in Freud's works in general. In my reading of *Dora* I want to show that neither Rose's and Gearhart's depoliticized theorizing nor Ramas' rather simplistic "feminist polemics" will really do. Feminists must neither reject theoretical discussion as "beyond feminist polemics" nor forget the ideological context of theory.

FRAGMENT OR WHOLE?

The first version of *Dora* was written in 1901. Freud entitled it "Dreams and Hysteria" and had the greatest ambitions for the text: this was his first great case history, and it was to continue and develop the work presented in *The Interpretation of Dreams*, published in the previous year. But Freud recalled *Dora* from his publisher and curiously enough delayed publication until 1905, the year of the *Three Essays on Sexuality*. Why would Freud hesitate for more than four years before deciding to publish *Dora?* According to Jacqueline Rose, this hesitation may have been because *Dora* was written in the period between the theory of the unconscious, developed in *The Interpretation of Dreams*, and the theory of sexuality, first expressed in the *Three Essays*. *Dora* would then mark the transition between these two theories, and Freud's hesitation in publishing the text suggests the theoretical hesitation within it. Jacqueline Rose may well be right in this supposition. It is at any rate evident that among Freud's texts *Dora* marks an unusual degree of uncertainty, doubt, and ambiguity.

This uncertainty is already revealed in the title of the work: the true title is not "Dora," but "Fragment of an Analysis of a Case of Hysteria." Freud lists three reasons for calling his text a fragment. First, the analytic results are fragmentary both because Dora interrupted the treatment before it was completed and because Freud did not write up the case history until after the treatment was over. The only exceptions to this are Dora's two dreams, which Freud took down immediately. The text we are reading, in other words, is constructed from fragmentary notes and Freud's fragmentary memory. Second, Freud insists on the fact that he has given an account only of the (incomplete) analytic *results* and not at all of the *process* of interpretation—that is to say, Freud willfully withholds the *technique of the analytic work*. To describe the analytic technique, Freud argues, would have led to "nothing but hopeless confusion" (*SE* 7:13; *P* 41; *C* 27). Finally, Freud stresses that no *one* case history can provide the answer to *all* the problems presented by hysteria: all case histories are in this sense incomplete answers to the problem they set out to solve.

It is of course perfectly normal to state, as Freud does here, the limitations of one's project in the preface to the finished work, but Freud does more than that. In his Prefatory Remarks to *Dora,* Freud seems positively obsessed with the incomplete status of his text. He returns to the subject again and again, either to excuse the fact that he is presenting a fragment or to express his longings for a *complete* text after all. His Prefatory Remarks oscillate constantly between the theme of fragmentation and the notion of totality. These two themes, however, are not presented as straight opposites. Having expressed his regrets that the case history is incomplete, he writes: "But its shortcomings are connected with the very circumstances which have made its publication possible. . . . I should not have known how to deal with the material involved in the history of a treatment which had lasted, perhaps, for a whole year" (*SE* 7:11; *P* 40; *C* 26). Freud here totally undermines any notion of a fundamental opposition between fragment and whole: it would have been impossible to write down a *complete* case history. The fragment can be presented as a complete book; the complete case history could not. Nevertheless, Freud insists on the fact that the fragment *lacks* something:

> In the face of the incompleteness of my analytic results, I had no choice but to follow the example of those discoverers whose good fortune it is to bring to the light of day after their long burial the priceless though mutilated relics of antiquity. I have restored what is missing, taking the best models known to me from other analyses; but like a conscientious archaeologist, I have not omitted to mention in each case where the authentic parts end and my construction begins. (*SE* 7:21; *P* 41; *C* 27)

Once again, Freud candidly admits that his results are incomplete—only to claim in the same breath that he has "restored what is missing": Freud's metaphors in this context are significant. Dora's story is compared to the "priceless though mutilated relics of antiquity," and Freud himself figures as an archeologist, digging relics out from the earth. His claim here is that when he adds something to the "mutilated relics," completeness is established *malgré tout*. But this new completeness is after all not quite complete. On the same page as the above quotation, Freud writes that the psychoanalytic technique (which he jealously retains for himself) does not by its nature lend itself to the creation of complete sequences: "Everything that has to do with the clearing-up of a particular symptom emerges piecemeal, woven into various contexts, and distributed over widely separated periods of time" (*SE* 7:12; *P* 41; *C* 27). The "completeness" achieved by Freud's supplementary conjectures is doubly incomplete: it consists of Dora's story (the "mutilated relics of antiquity"), to which Freud's own assumptions have been added. But Dora's story is not only a fragment: it is a fragment composed of information that has emerged "piecemeal, woven into various contexts, and distributed over widely separated periods of time." We must assume that it is Freud himself who has imposed a fictional coherence on Dora's story, in order to render the narrative readable. But Dora's story is in turn only one part of the finished work entitled "Fragment of an Analysis of a Case of Hysteria." The other part is supplemented by Freud. In itself Dora's story is too fragmentary; it is readable only when Freud supplies the necessary supplement. But that supplement is based on Freud's experience from other cases of hysteria, cases that must have been constructed in the same way as Dora's: by information provided "piecemeal, over widely separated periods of time." The fragment depends on the supplement, which depends on other fragments depending on other supplements, and so on ad infinitum.

We are, in other words, surprisingly close to Jacques Derrida's theories of the production of meaning as *"différance."*[4] According to Derrida, meaning can never be seized as presence: it is always deferred, constantly displaced onto the next element in the series, in a chain of signification that has no end, no transcendental signified that might provide the final anchor point for the production of sense. This, need one say, is not Freud's own *conscious* theory: he clings to his dream of "complete elucidation" (*SE* 7:24; *P* 54; *C* 39), refusing to acknowledge that according to his own account of the status of the *Dora* text, completeness is an unattainable illusion. Even when he insists strongly on the fragmentary status of his text, he always implies that completeness is within reach. He can, for instance, write, "If the work had been continued, we should no doubt have obtained the fullest possible enlightenment upon every particular of the case (*SE* 7:12; *P* 40; *C* 26). Freud's text oscillates endlessly between his desire for complete insight or knowledge and an unconscious realization (or fear) of the fragmentary, deferring status of knowledge itself.

TRANSFERENCE AND COUNTERTRANSFERENCE

We have seen that in his Prefatory Remarks Freud discloses that "Dora's story" *is* largely "Freud's story": he is the author, the one who has conjured a complete work from these analytic fragments. This in itself should alert the reader eager to discover Dora's own view of her case to the dangers of taking Freud's words too much at face value. His account of the analysis of Dora must instead be scanned with the utmost suspicion.

The better part of the Postcript is devoted to a discussion of the reasons why the analysis of Dora was at least in part a failure. Freud's main explanation is that he failed to discover the importance of the *transference* for the analysis; he did not discover in time that Dora was transferring the emotions she felt for Herr K. onto Freud himself. Psychoanalytic theory holds that transference is normal in the course of analysis, that it consists in the patient's transferring emotions for some other person onto the analyst, and that if the analyst, unaware of the transference, cannot counteract it, the analysis will in consequence go awry.

Freud adds this information in this Postscript. But if we are to grasp what is being acted out between Freud and Dora, it is important to keep in mind from the outset this transference on Dora's part from Herr K. to Freud. Transference, however, is something the patient does to the analyst. Freud does not mention at all the opposite phenomenon, *countertransference,* which consists in the analyst's transferring his or her own unconscious emotions onto the patient. Jacques Lacan has discussed precisely this problem in *Dora* in an article entitled "Intervention sur le transfert."[5] According to Lacan, Freud unconsciously identifies with Herr K. in his relationship to Dora, which makes him (Freud) far too interested in Dora's alleged love for Herr K. and effectively blind to any other explanation of her problems. Thus the countertransference contributes decisively to the failure of Dora's analysis.

The fact of transference and countertransference between Freud and Dora considerably complicates the task of the *Dora* reader. Freud's attempts to posit himself as the neutral, scientific observer who is merely noting down his observations and reflections can no longer be accepted. The archeologist must be suspected of having mutilated the relics he finds. We must remember that Freud's version of the case is colored not only by his own unconscious countertransference but also by the fact that he signally fails to notice the transference in Dora, and therefore systematically misinterprets her transference symptoms throughout the text. This, oddly, is something the reader is not told until the "Postscript."

Freud's interpretation of Dora's case can be summarized as follows. Dora develops hysterical symptoms because she represses sexual desire. But her case has an added, oedipal dimension: one must suppose that Dora originally desired her father, but since her father disappointed her by starting an affair with Frau K., Dora now pretends to hate him. Herr K. represents the father for Dora, particularly because he is also Frau K.'s husband. Dora's repression of her sexual desire for Herr K. is therefore at once a hysterical reaction (repression of sexual desire) *and* an oedipal reaction (rejection of the father through rejection of Herr K.). Based on this interpretation, Freud's treatment of Dora consists in repeated attempts to get her to admit her repressed desire for Herr K., a "confession" Dora resists as best she can.

We have already seen that, according to Lacan, the analysis failed because of Freud's unconscious identification with Herr K. Since Dora is at the same time identifying Freud with Herr K., the result is inevitably that she must experience Freud's insistence on the necessity of acknowledging her desire for Herr K. as a repetition of Herr K.'s attempt to elicit sexual favors from her. In the end she rejects Freud in the same way she rejected Herr K.—by giving him two weeks' notice. Herr K. had earlier had an affair with the governess of his children, and Dora felt greatly insulted at being courted like a servant by the same man. Her revenge is to treat both Freud and Herr K. as servants in return.

But Freud's incessant identification with Herr K., the rejected lover, leads to other interesting aspects of the text. One of the most important episodes in the study is Freud's interpretation of Herr K.'s attempt to kiss Dora, then fourteen, after having tricked her into being alone with him in his office. Freud writes that Herr K.

> suddenly clasped the girl to him and pressed a kiss upon her lips. This was surely just the situation to call up a distinct feeling of sexual excitement in a girl of fourteen who had never before been approached. But Dora had at that moment a violent feeling of disgust, tore herself free from the man, and hurried past him to the staircase and from there to the street door. (*SE* 7:28; *P* 59; *C* 43)

At this moment in the text Freud is completely in the grip of his countertransference: he must at all costs emphasize that Dora's reaction was abnormal and writes that "the behaviour of this child of fourteen was already entirely and completely hysterical" (*SE* 7:28; *P* 59; *C* 44). Her reaction was hysterical because she was already repressing sexual desire: "Instead of the genital sensation which would certainly have been felt by a healthy girl in such circumstances, Dora was overcome by . . . disgust" (*SE* 7:29; *P* 60; *C* 44). It is, of course, resplendently clear to any scientific observer that any normal girl of fourteen would be overwhelmed by desire when a middle-aged man "suddenly clasps her to him" in a lonely spot.

Freud then links Dora's feeling of disgust to *oral* impulses and goes on to interpret as a "displacement" Dora's statement that she clearly felt the pressure from the upper part of Herr K.'s body against her own. What she really felt, according to Freud, and what aroused such strong oral disgust, was the pressure of Herr K.'s erect penis. The thought of this unmentionable organ was then repressed, and the feeling of pressure displaced from the lower to the upper part of the body. The oral disgust is then related to Dora's habit of thumb-sucking as a child, and Freud connects the oral satisfaction resulting from this habit to Dora's nervous cough. He interprets the cough (irritation of oral cavity and throat) as a revealing symptom of Dora's sexual fantasies: she must be fantasizing a scene where sexual satisfaction is obtained by using the mouth (*per os*, as Freud puts it) (*SE* 7:48; *P* 81; *C* 65), and this scene is one that takes place between Frau K. and Dora's father.

Having said as much, Freud spends the next few pages defending himself against accusations of using too foul a language with his patients. These passages could be read as betraying a certain degree of unconscious tension in Freud himself, but it is enough to point out here that he argues his way from exhortations to tolerance to the high social status of "the perversion which is the most repellent to us, the sensual love of a man for a man" (*SE* 7:50; *P* 93; *C* 67) in ancient Greece, before returning to Dora's oral fantasy and making it plain that what he had in mind was fellatio, or "sucking at the male organ" (*SE* 7:51; *P* 85; *C* 68). It would not be difficult to detect in Freud a defensive reaction-formation in this context, since on the next page he feels compelled to allude to "this excessively repulsive and perverted phantasy of sucking at a penis" (*SE* 7:52; *P* 86; *C* 69). It is little wonder that he feels the need to defend himself against the idea of fellatio, since it is more than probable that the fantasy exists, not in Dora's mind, but in his alone. Freud has informed us that Dora's father was impotent, and assumes this to be the basis of Dora's "repulsive and perverted phantasy." According to Freud, the father cannot manage penetration, so Frau K. must perform fellatio instead. But as Lacan has pointed out, this argument reveals an astonishing lack of logic on Freud's part. In the case of male impotence, the man is obviously much more likely, *faute de mieux,* to perform cunnilingus. As Lacan writes: "Everyone knows that cunnilingus is the artifice most commonly adopted by 'men of means' whose powers begin to abandon them." It is in this logical flaw that Freud's countertransference is seen at its strongest. The illogicality reveals his own unconscious wish for gratification, a gratification Freud's unconscious alter ego, Herr K., might obtain if only Dora would admit her desire for him.

Freud's countertransference blinds him to the possibility that Dora's hysteria may be due to the repression of desire, not for Herr K., but for his wife, Frau K. A fatal lack of insight into the transferential process prevents Freud from discovering Dora's homosexuality early enough. Dora's condition as a victim of male dominance here becomes starkly visible. She is not only a pawn in the game between Herr K. and her father; her doctor joins the male team and untiringly tries to ascribe to her desires she does not have and to ignore the ones she does have.

PATRIARCHAL PREJUDICES

Freud's oppressive influence on Dora does not, however, stem only from the countertransference. There are also more general ideological tendencies to sexism at work in his text. Freud, for instance, systematically refuses to consider female sexuality as an active, independent drive. Again and again he exhorts Dora to accept herself as an object for Herr K. Every time Dora reveals active sexual desires, Freud interprets them away, either by assuming that Dora is expressing masculine identification (when she fantasizes about female genitals, Freud instantly assumes that she wants to penetrate them) or by supposing that she desires to be penetrated by the male (Dora's desire for Frau K. is interpreted as her desire to be in Frau K.'s place in order to gain access to Herr K.). His position is self-contradictory: he is one of the first to acknowledge the existence of sexual desire in women, and at the same time he renders himself incapable of seeing it as more than the impulse to become passive recipients for male desire. Lacan assumes precisely the same attitude when he states that the problem for Dora (and all women) is that she "must accept herself as the object of male desire" (Lacan) and that this is the reason for Dora's adoration of Frau K.

Feminists cannot help feeling relieved when Dora finally dismisses Freud like another servant. It is tempting to read Dora's hysterical symptoms, as do Cixous and Clément, as a silent revolt against male power over women's bodies and women's language. But at the same time it is disconcerting to see how inefficient Dora's revolt turned out to be. Felix Deutsch describes Dora's tragic destiny in an article written in 1957. She continued to develop various hysterical symptoms, made life unbearable for her family, and grew to resemble her mother (whom Freud dismissed as a typical case of "housewife psychosis"). According to Deutsch, Dora tortured her husband throughout their marriage; he concluded that "her marriage had served only to cover up her distaste of men" (see essay 1). Dora suffers continuously from psychosomatic constipation and dies from cancer of the colon. Deutsch concludes, "Her death . . . seemed a blessing to those who were close to her. She had been, as my informant phrased it, one of the most repulsive hysterics he had ever met."

It may be gratifying to see the young, proud Dora as a radiant example of feminine revolt (as does Cixous); but we should not forget the image of the old, nagging, whining, and complaining Dora she later becomes, achieving nothing. Hysteria is not, *pace* Hélène Cixous, the incarnation of the revolt of women forced to silence but rather a declaration of defeat, the realization that there is no other way out. Hysteria is, as Catherine Clément perceives, a cry for help when defeat becomes real, when the woman sees that she is efficiently gagged and chained to her feminine role.

Now if the hysterical woman is gagged and chained, Freud posits himself as her liberator. And if the emancipatory project of psychoanalysis fails in the case of Dora, it is because Freud the liberator happens also to be, objectively, on the side of oppression. He is a male in patriarchal society, and moreover not just any male but an educated bourgeois male, incarnating *malgré lui* patriarchal values. His own emancipatory project profoundly conflicts with his political and social role as an oppressor of women.

The most telling instance of this deeply unconscious patriarchal ideology in *Dora* is to be found in Freud's obsession with the sources of his patient's sexual information. After stressing the impossibility of tracing the sources of Dora's sexual information (*SE* 7:31; *P* 62; *C* 46), Freud nevertheless continually returns to the subject, suggesting alternately that the source may have been books belonging to a former governess (*SE* 7:36; *P* 68; *C* 52), Mantegazza's *Physiology of Love* (*SE* 7:62; *P* 97; *C* 80), or an encyclopedia (*SE* 7:99; *P 140; C* 120). He finally realizes that there must have been an *oral* source of information, in addition to the avid reading of forbidden books, then sees, extremely belatedly, that the oral source must have been none other than the beloved Frau K.

The one hypothesis that Freud does not entertain is that the source of oral information may have been Dora's mother—the mother who is traditionally charged with the sexual education of the daughters. This omission is wholly symptomatic of Freud's treatment of Dora's mother. Although he indicates Dora's identification with her mother (*SE* 7:75; *P* 111; *C* 93), he nevertheless strongly insists that Dora had withdrawn completely from her mother's influence (*SE* 7:23; *P* 50; *C* 38). Dora's apparent hatred of her mother is mobilized as evidence for this view.

But Freud ought to know better than to accept a daughter's hatred of her mother as an inevitable consequence of the mother's objective unlikableness ("housewife's psychosis"). Even his own oedipal explanation of Dora's rejection of Herr K. should contribute to a clearer understanding of the mother's importance for Dora. Oedipally speaking, Dora would be seen as the mother's rival in that competition for the father's love, but this rivalry also implies the necessity of identifying with the mother: the daughter must become like the mother in order to be loved by the father. Freud notes that Dora is behaving like a jealous wife and that this behavior shows that "she was clearly putting herself in her mother's place" (*SE* 7:56; *P* 90; *C* 73), but he draws no further conclusions from these observations. He also points out that

Dora identifies with Frau K., her father's mistress, but is still quite content to situate her mainly in relation to her father and Herr K. He fails to see that Dora is caught up in an ambivalent relationship to her mother and an idealizing and identifying relationship to Frau K., the other mother-figure in this text. Freud's patriarchal prejudices force him to ignore relationships between women and instead center all his attention on relationships with men. This grievous underestimation of the importance of other women for Dora's psychic development contributes decisively to the failure of the analysis and the cure—not least in that it makes Freud unaware of the *preoedipal* causes for Dora's hysteria. Maria Ramas writes: "By Freud's own admission, the deepest level of meaning of hysterical symptoms is not a thwarted desire for the father, but a breakthrough of the prohibited desire for the mother."

SEXUALITY AND EPISTEMOLOGY

Freud's particular interest in the sources of Dora's sexual information does not, however, merely reveal that for as long as possible he avoids considering oral relations between women as such a source; it also indicates that Freud overestimates the importance of this question. There is nothing in Dora's story to indicate that a successful analysis depends on the elucidation of this peripheral problem. Why then would Freud be so obsessed by these sources of knowledge?

First, because he himself desires total knowledge: his aim is nothing less than the *complete elucidation* of Dora, despite his insistence on the fragmentary nature of his material. The absence of information on this one subject is thus tormenting, since it so obviously ruins the dream of completeness. But such a desire for total, absolute knowledge exposes a fundamental assumption in Freud's epistemology. Knowledge for Freud is a finished, closed whole. Possession of knowledge means possession of power. Freud, the doctor, is curiously proud of his hermeneutical capacities. After having interpreted Dora's fingering of her little purse as an admission of infantile masturbation, he writes with evident satisfaction:

When I set myself the task of bringing to light what human beings keep hidden within them, not by the compelling power of hypothesis, but by observing what they say and what they show, I thought the task was a harder one than it really is. He that has eyes to see and ears to hear may convince himself that no mortal can keep a secret. If his lips are silent, he chatters with his finger tips; betrayal oozes out of him at every pore. And thus the task of making conscious the most hidden recesses of the mind is one which it is quite possible to accomplish. (*SE* 7:77–8; *P* 114; *C* 96)

Freud in other words possesses powers more compelling than those of hypnosis. He is the one who discloses and unlocks secrets; he is Oedipus solving the Sphinx's riddle. But like Oedipus he is ravaged by a terrible anxiety: the fear of castration. If Freud cannot solve Dora's riddle, the unconscious punishment for this failure will be castration. In this struggle for the possession of knowledge, a knowledge that is power, Dora reveals herself both as Freud's alter ego and as his rival. She possesses the secret Freud is trying to discover. At this point we must suspect Freud of countertransference to Dora: he identifies with the hysterical Dora in the search for information about sexual matters. Freud has his own secret, as Dora has hers: the analytic technique, which, as we have seen, cannot be exposed without causing "total confusion." Freud jealously keeps his secret, as Dora keeps hers: her homosexual desire for Frau K.

But since Dora is a woman, and a rather formidable one at that, a young lady who hitherto has had only scorn for the incompetent (and, surely, impotent) doctors who have treated her so far, she becomes a threatening rival for Freud. If he does not win the fight for knowledge, he will also be revealed as incompetent/impotent, his compelling powers will be reduced to nothing, he will be castrated. If Dora wins the knowledge game, her model for knowledge will emerge victorious, and Freud's own model will be destroyed. Freud here finds himself between Scylla and Charybdis: if he identifies with Dora in the search for knowledge, he becomes a woman, that is to say, castrated; but if he chooses to cast her as his rival, he *must* win out, or the punishment will be castration.

The last point (that the punishment in case of defeat will be castration) requires further explanation. We have seen that Dora's sources of knowledge have been characterized as female, oral, and scattered. Freud, on the contrary, presents his knowledge as something that creates a unitary whole. In both cases we are discussing sexual knowledge. But Freud's own paradigmatic example of the desire for sexual knowledge is the sexual curiosity in children, and Freud's most important text on this topic is *Little Hans*. Moving from *Dora* to *Little Hans*, the reader is struck by this remarkable difference in tone between the two texts. The five-year-old little Hans, straining to understand the mysteries of sexuality, is strongly encouraged in his epistemophilia (Freud's own word, from *Three Essays on Sexuality*). Freud never ceases to express his admiration for the intelligence of the little boy, in such laudatory statements as, "Here the little boy was displaying a really unusual degree of clarity" (*SE* 10:44; *P* 206), or "Little Hans has by a bold stroke taken the conduct of the analysis into his own hands. By means of a brilliant symptomatic act . . ." (*SE* 10:86; *P* 246). This tone is far removed from Freud's stern admonitions of Dora, his continuous *et tu quoque* ripostes to her interpretation of her own situation.

Why this differential treatment? It is arguable that in *Little Hans* Freud equates the desire for knowledge and the construction of theories with the desire to discover the role of the penis in procreation. The penis, in other words, becomes the epistemological object par excellence for Freud. But if this is so, knowledge and theory must be conceptualized as whole, rounded, finished—just like the penis. Little Hans becomes in this sense a penis for Freud. He is both a pleasurable object to be studied, a source of excitation and enthusiasm, *and* Freud's double: a budding sexual theoretician emerging to confirm Freud's own epistemological activities. But where Little Hans confirms, Dora threatens. Her knowledge cannot be conceptualized as a whole; it is dispersed and has been assembled piecemeal from feminine sources. Dora's epistemological model becomes the female genitals, which in Freud's vision emerge as unfinished, diffuse, and fragmentary; they cannot add up to a complete whole and must therefore be perceived as castrated genitals. If Freud were to accept Dora's epistemological model, it would be tantamout to rejecting the penis as the principal symbol for human desire for knowledge, which again would mean accepting castration.

Freud's masculine psyche therefore perceives Dora as more fundamentally threatening than he can consciously express. Instead, his fear of epistemological castration manifests itself in various disguises: in his obsessive desire to discover the sources of Dora's knowledge, and in his oddly intense discussion of the fragmentary status of the *Dora* text. To admit that there are holes in one's knowledge is tantamount to transforming the penis to a hole, that is to say, to transforming the man into a woman. Holes, empty spaces, open areas are at all cost to be avoided; and with this in mind we can discern further layers of meaning in the passage quoted earlier:

> In the face of the incompleteness of my analytic results, I had no choice but to follow the example of those discoverers whose good fortune it is to bring to the light of day after their long burial the priceless though mutilated relics of antiquity. I have restored what is missing. (*SE* 7:12; *P* 41; *C* 27)

"The priceless though mutilated relics of antiquity" are not only Dora's story: they are Dora herself, her genitals and the feminine epistemological model. Freud makes sure that the message here is clear: "mutilated" is his usual way of describing the effect of castration, and "priceless" also means just what it says: price-less, without value. For how can there be value when the valuable piece has been cut off?[6] The relics are mutilated, the penis has been cut. Freud's task is therefore momentous: he must "restore what is missing"; his penis must fill the epistemological hole represented by Dora.

But such a task can only be performed by one who possesses what is missing. And this is precisely what Freud occasionally doubts in his text: the fear of castration is also the fear of discovering that one has already been castrated. Freud's hesitation in *Dora* between insisting on completeness and admitting fragmentary status indicates that in his text the penis is playing a kind of *fort-da* game with its author (now you have it, now you don't).[7] Freud's book about Dora is the narrative of an intense power struggle between two protagonists—a struggle in which the male character's virility is at stake and in which he by no means always has the upper hand.

When Dora dismisses Freud like a servant, she paradoxically rescues him from further epistemological insecurity. He is left, then, the master of the *writing* of Dora. And even though his text bears the scars of the struggle between him and his victim, it is a victorious Freud who publishes it. Dora dismissed him, but Freud got his revenge: Dora was the name Freud's own sister, Rosa, had foisted on her maid in place of her real one, which also was Rosa (*The Psychopathology of Everyday Life, SE* 6:241). So Ida Bauer, in a bitter historical irony, was made famous under the name of a servant after all.

Freud's epistemology is clearly phallocentric. The male is the bearer of knowledge; he alone has the power to penetrate woman and text; woman's role is to let herself be penetrated by such truth. Such epistemological phallocentrism is by no means specifically Freudian; on the contrary, it has so far enjoyed universal sway in our patriarchal civilization, and one could hardly expect Freud to emerge untouched by it. It is politically important, however, to point out that this pathological division of knowledge into masculine totality and feminine fragment is completely mystifying and mythological. There is absolutely no evidence for the actual existence of two such gender-determined sorts of knowledge, to be conceptualized as parallel to the shapes of human genitals. Dora can be perceived as the bearer of feminine epistemology in the study only because Freud selected her as his opponent in a war over cognition, creating her as his symbolic antagonist. To champion Dora's "feminine values" means meekly accepting Freud's own definitions of masculine and feminine. Power always creates its own definitions, and this is particularly true of the distinctions between masculine and feminine constructed by patriarchal society. Nowhere is patriarchal ideology to be seen more clearly than in the definition of the feminine as the negative of the masculine—and this is precisely how Freud defines Dora and the "feminine" epistemology she is supposed to represent.

To undermine this phallocentric epistemology means to expose its lack of "natural" foundation. In the case of *Dora,* however, we have been able to do this only because of Freud's own theories of femininity and sexuality. The attack upon phallocentrism must come from within, since there can be no "outside," no space where true femininity, untainted by patriarchy, can be kept intact for us to discover. We can only destroy the mythical and mystifying constructions of patriarchy by using its own weapons. We have no others.

Notes

1. Hélène Cixous and Catherine Clément, *La jeune née* (Paris: Editions 10/18, 1975).

2. Hélène Cixous, *Portrait de Dora* (Paris: Editions des femmes, 1976). This play has been translated by Sarah Burd in *Diacritics* (Spring 1983), pp. 2–32. Another translation, by Anita Barrows, has been published in *Benmussa Directs* (London: Calder, 1979; Dallas: Riverrun Press, 1979).

3. Maria Ramas cut this passage from the shortened version of her essay published in this book. The full version is in *Feminist Studies*, (Fall 1980), 6(3):500—Editors' note.

4. Jacques Derrida, *Marges de la philosophie* (Paris: Minuit, 1972).

5. Jacques Lacan, *Écrits* (Paris: Seuil, 1966), p. 224. See Jacqueline Rose's translation of "Intervention sur le transfert," essay 4 of this book.

6. Freud always assumes that castration means the cutting off of the penis. This is quite odd; not so much because real castration consists in the cutting off of the testicles, but because he nowhere refers to this discrepancy between his own definition of castration and the real practice.

7. The *fort-da* game is the game in which the child, by rejecting and retrieving a toy, enacts the absence and presence of the mother. *Fort-da* means roughly *"here-gone."*

9. Keys to Dora

JANE GALLOP

In 1976 a book was published in France, on the cover of which we read: "Portrait de Dora/de Hélène Cixous/des femmes." These three lines are repeated on the title page, but there "des femmes" is followed by an address—2 rue de la Roquette 75011 Paris—for it is the name of a publishing house linked with the woman's group called "Psychoanalysis and Politics." As the name of a press, "des femmes" appears on many books, but it seems particularly resonant on this cover, where it occasions the third occurrence of the preposition "de" (of, from). The unusual inclusion of a "de" before the author's name works to draw the heroine Dora, the author, Hélène Cixous, as well as the press's name, that is "women," into a circuit of substitution embodied in the grammatical structure of apposition. The portrait of Dora is also a portrait of Hélène Cixous is also a portrait of women (in general).

According to the dictionary, a "portrait" is a "representation of a real person." "Representation" has a theatrical as well as a visual sense, and Cixous's text is a play, a theatrical script. But "portrait" also has an interesting figurative sense. The dictionary *(Le Petit Robert)* gives the following example from Balzac: "Virginie était tout le *portrait de* sa mère" (emphasis mine), as we say in English, "Virginia was the (spit-

This text appears as ch. 9 of Jane Gallop, *The Daughter's Seduction: Feminism and Psychoanalysis* (London: Macmillan, 1982; Ithaca: Cornell University Press, 1982).

ting) image of her mother." "Portrait" itself leads us not only to representation in the visual and theatrical senses, but to re-presentation, replication, the substitutability of one woman for another.

Dora is Freud's Dora, the name Freud gives to the heroine of his "Fragment of an Analysis of a Case of Hysteria," published in 1905. In this case history, Freud writes of Dora's complaint that she is being used as an "object of barter." Dora protests that her father has handed her over to his friend in exchange for that friend's wife. Freud does not disagree with Dora's inference but merely states that this is not a "formal agreement" between the two men but one that the men do without being conscious of it. Dora and Freud have discovered a fragment of the general structure that thirty years later Claude Lévi-Strauss will call elementary kinship structures, that is, the exchange of women between men. Lévi-Strauss' formulation of this general system of exchange is structuralism's major contribution to feminist theory.

In another book, *La jeune née,* which has become a major text of French feminist theory, Cixous writes, "I am what Dora would have been if the history of women *[histoire des femmes]* had begun."[1] The *histoire* (history, story) that intervenes is *des femmes,* taking that phrase as both objective and subjective genitive. The cover of *Portrait* imposes a double reading of the "de" in "des femmes," since it follows two opposing uses of the preposition. The history of women must also be a history by women, women making their own history. *Histoire des femmes:* a story coming from women, a story published by the press *des femmes* (what Anglophone feminists call "herstory") alters the identification between Dora and Cixous. By passing through the terms "des femmes," whose generality appropriately designates a press, that which places words in general circulation, the triple identification saves Cixous from being simply another Dora, as Dora was rather than as she "would have been."

La jeune née is comprised of three sections: the first by Catherine Clément, the second by Hélène Cixous, the third an unprepared, unedited dialogue between the two. Throughout *La jeune née* the hysteric, particularly Dora, functions as an insistent question the two women writers are asking: Is she a heroine or a victim?

At the beginning of the book, Clément declares that the role of the hysteric is ambiguous: she both contests and conserves (p. 13). The hysteric contests inasmuch as she "undoes family ties, introduces perturbation into the orderly unfolding of daily life, stirs up magic in apparent reason" (pp. 13–14). But the hysteric's contestation is contained and co-opted, and, like any victory of the familiar, the familial over the heterogeneous and alien, this containment serves to strengthen the family. "Every hysteric ends up inuring the others to her symptoms, and the family closes up once more around her" (p. 14). The family assimilates her otherness, and like an amoeba, finds its single cell revitalized, stronger than before.

Thus upon its first appearance the question of the hysteric's role seems answered, resolved into an irresolvable but stable and determinable ambiguity. Yet as the book continues, the ambiguity defined by Clément seems not so stable, not so easy to declare and accept as such. Just as the hysteric perturbs the orderly unfolding of family life, might she not likewise disturb the position of authorial mastery in this book? This cannot be considered a failing in a book where the desirability of a masterful authorial discourse is itself called into question. But to be unseated by hysteria is not the same as to give up intentionally one's masterful position. The reasonable, forceful, clever position for the two women theorists is to assume the inevitability of ambiguity. To choose ambiguity is to choose to give up one's masterful position, is simply a ruse toward a more resilient mastery. Yet rather than assume the ambiguity, the two writers themselves become polarized as advocates of *either* the hysteric as contesting *or* the hysteric as conserving.

During a discussion of the hysteric's role, Clément says to Cixous, "Listen, you really like Dora, but as for me, she has never seemed to me to be a revolutionary heroine." To which Cixous replies, "I don't give a damn about Dora, I don't fetishize her. She is the name of a certain disturbing force which means that the little circus no longer runs" (p. 289). Cixous's testy, defensive reply, "I don't give a damn. . . . I don't fetishize her" picks up, with perhaps hysterical hypersensitivity, the implicit and personal accusation in Clément's "Listen, you really like Dora, but as for me." Clément needs to make her position clear, to distinguish herself from Cixous, to distinguish between "you" and "me," and, more urgently, to distinguish herself from Cixous's identification with Dora.

Whereas Cixous can write, "The hysterics are my sisters" (p. 184), in the same book Clément declares, "Physically [the hysterics] are no longer . . . and if someone dresses up like one, it is a disguise. They are obsolete figures. . . . I really liked them, but they no longer exist" (p. 111). Clément writes, "I really liked them," in the past tense, whereas she later says to Cixous, "You really like Dora" in the present tense. The disagreement seems to be a struggle to keep the hysteric an "obsolete figure," to keep the hysterical identification in the past. To understand more fully this outburst—"I don't give a damn. . . . I don't fetishize her"—let us follow the argument in the pages immediately preceding this moment:

Cixous asserts, "It is very difficult to block this sort of person who leaves you no peace, who makes permanent war against you" (p. 287). War functions in Cixous's section of the book as a positive value, necessary for transformation. If the hysteric makes "permanent war," leaves "no peace," then she must be safely ensconced on the side of contestation, unambiguously nonassimilable. But to Cixous's assertion, Clément replies: "Yes, that introduces dissension, but it in no way makes anything burst; that does not *disperse* the bourgeois family, which only exists through her dissension, which only holds together in the possibility or the reality of its own disturbance, always re-closable, always re-closed" (p. 287; Clément's italics). The contesting hysteric is thus necessary to the family cell and serves a conservative function. Rather than seeing the hysteric's role as ambiguous, Clément now argues that it is only deluded, co-opted rebellion. She may appear to disturb, but the hysteric actually provides an opportunity for the family to revitalize itself through the assimilation of something outside itself. She feeds the family machine. A heroine for Cixous, Dora is only a victim for Clément.

According to Clément, the difference between those whose violence is reassimilable and those whose contestation is effective lies in the attainment of "symbolic inscription" (p. 288). The Lacanian term "symbolic" that Clément uses here is in contradistinction to the term "imaginary." Whereas the imaginary is a closed circle, the "symbolic" opens out into a generalized exchange. Lacan takes the term "symbolic" from Lévi-Strauss. Lévi-Strauss's kinship structures belong to the symbolic order, whereas Dora's and Freud's fragment of those structures remain within the particular family as a perverse exception. Mirroring, one-to-one identification typifies the imaginary register. Following Clément's standard of "symbolic inscription," we can see that Cixous's identification with Dora is saved from the circular delusions and powerlessness of the imaginary because it passes through the third term on the cover, passes through the press *des femmes.* Once published, the scandal can no longer be contained within the family. Publication "disperses," to use the word Clément emphasizes. The circle of the family is broken; the cell walls burst.

For Clément, Dora does not pass into "symbolic inscription," and so Dora's outbursts burst nothing. According to Clément: "Raising a ruckus, causing a crisis, perturbing familial relations, that is re-closable." But Cixous responds, "And it is that very force which works in the dismantling of structures. . . . Dora broke something." Clément replies: "I don't think so" (pp. 288–89).

The disagreement turns around the question of whether something is broken or not, open or closed. In a footnote to the Dora case, Freud writes: "The question whether a woman is 'open' or 'shut' can naturally not be a matter of indifference" *(SE 7:67n; C 84n.).* The question of open or shut cannot be left undecided, ambiguous. Clément has articulated the question of whether a woman contests or conserves around the distinction open or shut. Although Clément begins by defining the hysteric's position as ambiguous, once it is tied to the question "open or shut," that ambiguity becomes intolerable; it must be decided. As in Freud's footnote, what is at stake is a woman's honor. Is Dora compromised or not?

Still and all, from Freud's footnote to *La jeune née,* things have changed. For Clément and Cixous, the heroine is she who has broken something. In the 1975 text, compromise attaches to the woman who is shut up, whereas in Freud's context it is the open woman whose honor is compromised. This is not a simple reversal of values: a shift in grammatical position alters the opposition in a manner more complex than reversal. In Freud's question the woman is, in either case, grammatically passive: she remains passively "shut" or she is "open" through an outside agent, a man. But in *La jeune née,* that which cannot be "a matter of indifference" involves a difference in the woman's grammatical position. Does she "open" the family, or is she "shut" by it? The 1975 question "open" or "shut" includes a second question, the question of woman as agent or patient. In Freud's text she can only be patient, in fact, Dr. Freud's patient. But just as the agent of the "Portrait" (de Hélène Cixous) can identify/be identified with the patient of the "Portrait" (de Dora), the advent of the "histoire des femmes," the case history of and by women, gives the woman the agency to open, allows her to do more than patiently wait for a determination of what can "naturally" not be a matter of indifference.

The distinction "open" or "shut" matters in *La jeune née*. Cixous's section is entitled "Sorties," which can be translated as "exits, outlets, escapes, holidays, outings, sallies, sorties," also "outbursts, attacks, tirades." Let us remark especially the warlike and the hysterical senses ("attack"), but in general there is a sense of exits, openings, escapes from enclosures. Also, the disagreement between Clément and Cixous is located in a published dialogue. The choice to publish a "dissension," to bring it to "symbolic inscription," is the choice to leave it open, not to try to reassimilate it, to shut it up, or to keep it within the family. Freud's open-and-shut footnote specifically refers to Dora's concern over whether a door is locked or not, which comes up in her associations to the "first dream" of the case. Freud's footnote extends the door metaphor: "The question whether a woman is 'open' or 'shut' can naturally not be a matter of indifference. It is well known, too, what sort of 'key' effects the opening in such a case." Cixous has Freud speak these two sentences to Dora in the play. Dora says, "When I wanted . . . to close myself in to rest, no more key! I am sure it was Mr. K. who had taken it away." Freud then pronounces the two sentences, to which Dora replies, "I was 'sure' you would say that!" (pp. 48–49). The two "sure's"—the second one in quotation marks, apparently a quote from the first one—connect Dora's certainty about Herr K.'s culpable intentions and her certainty about Freud, bringing out her substitution of Freud for Herr K. in the transference.

Later in his text on Dora, Freud writes, "Sexuality is the key to the problem of the psychoneuroses and of the neuroses in general. No one who disdains the key will ever be able to unlock the door" (*SE* 7:115; *C* 136). That the "well-known," "natural" sexual imagery of the footnote should recur in Freud's discussion of his own enterprise seems to bear out Dora's suspicion that Freud is somehow in the position of Herr K. Both hold the key and are threatening to unlock the door.

Portrait's framing of the footnote sentences with Dora's two "sure's" also brings out the smug certitude of Freud's "naturally" and his "well-known." Is this not the worst sort of vulgar, predictable "Freudian" interpretation? The predictability of Freud's line about keys offends Dora by denying the specificity of her signifiers (by not attending to her but merely applying general formulas) in the same way that she is offended by Herr K.'s beginning his declaration of love with what she knew were the same words he had used to seduce a governess. What woman wants to be opened by a skeleton key?

Cixous says of the case of Dora, "I immediately operated a reading that was probably not centered as Freud wanted it to be. . . . I read it as a fiction" (*La jeune née*, p. 272). Freud begins the case history with instructions as to how it ought to be read. It ought to be read scientifically; but even as he writes it, he is aware there will be those readers who pervert (Cixous would say "decenter") his intentions, who read it for pleasure. From Freud's Preface to the Dora case: "I am aware that—in this city, at least—there are many physicians who (revolting though it may seem) choose to read a case history of this kind not as a contribution to the psychopathology of neuroses, but as a *roman à clef* designed for their private delectation" (*SE* 7:9; *C* 23). The English translation borrows a French expression to render Freud's "*Schlüsselroman,*" literally, "key-novel." The vulgar, perverse reading Freud fears would entail looking for "keys" in his text, as one would in a novel (Cixous's "fiction").

Somehow the base, the vulgar in the Dora case is connected three times to "keys": (1) the vulgar, "revolting" reading looks for keys (*SE* 7:9; *C* 23); (2) Freud's footnote refers to the "well-known" symbolism of keys (*SE* 7:67; *C* 84), thus himself giving a common, vulgar interpretation; and (3) finally, we are told in the Postface that "sexuality is the key" (*SE* 7:115; *C* 136). Freud knows that many will "disdain" this key, that is, find it "revolting," vulgar, below them. Is not his disgust at his vulgar readers, who read for their own "delectation," a similar gesture of contempt for the sexual, particularly for the perverse—those components of sexuality that simply give pleasure as opposed to work for reproduction (cf. "read not as a contribution but for their delectation")? Perhaps Cixous's decentering, perverse reading of Dora as a fiction of keys recovers the "revolting," scandalous force of Freud's discovery of infantile, perverse sexuality.

It is interesting to note that the kind of reading Freud expected and dreaded from the physicians, "of this city, at least," must be represented in the English translation by a French phrase, *roman à clef.* In the eyes of the traditional English-speaking psychoanalytic community, the reading of Freud currently practiced in France is likewise inappropriate and unscientific. The French are reading Freud literarily, as if it were a novel, paying attention to the letter of his text, to such trivial details as the repeated appearance of the word *Schlüssel.* The inappropriateness of French Freud, however, seems to rejoin some original Viennese reading. The original German text did not need the French phrase. Perhaps, for those of us who read Freud in English, a French detour is necessary in order to recover the original, scandalous Viennese reading, in order not to lose the "key."

A French detour may be literally—that is, *à la lettre*—necessary. The English translator chooses to use the French *détour* rather than the English *detour* for the German *Umwege,* that is, chooses to include the acute accent, in the following sentence from the Dora case: "The dream, in short, is one of the *détours by which repression can be evaded*" (*SE* 7:15; *C* 29). Freud's German sentence has no italics; they originate in the English translation, as if this sentence were of particular importance to the English text, the English context. According to certain French psychoanalysts, particularly Lacan, English and American psychoanalysis has repressed the unconscious out of psychoanalysis. In that context the *détour,* the French detour, a detour through the French reading of Freud, *à la lettre,* is perhaps a means, a hope for evading repression, the repression of what is "revolting," that is, original in Freud.

There is another equally apt occasion when the English translator finds it necessary to render Freud's German with a French phrase. Freud states that "the determination of Dora's symptoms is far too specific for it to be possible to expect a frequent recurrence of the same accidental aetiology" (*SE* 7:40; *C* 56). This assertion puts into doubt the value of publishing this case history, its value as "a contribution." "Have we not merely allowed ourselves to become the victims of a *jeu d'espirit?*" asks Freud in the English translation. The French is occasioned by the German *Spiel des Witzes.* Anglophone psychoanalysis has often dismissed the current Parisian equivalent as unserious word play, mere punning. The German word *Witz* can be construed as an allusion to *Jokes and Their Relation to the Unconscious (Der Witz . . .),* published by Freud in the same year as the Dora case. The French have paid great attention to this jokebook as one of the best illustrations that what Freud discovered is an unconscious structured like a language.

Freud is here discussing the problem of the "skeleton key," the interpretation that fits many similar cases. Freud's radical discovery was the specificity expressed in every symptom. Yet the fate of psychoanalysis in the English-speaking countries, where it achieved such popularity, was to become a set system of interpretation, a ready-made symbolism to be applied to many cases, giving it an obvious market value, quieting the very doubt Freud expresses here. Again, it may be necessary to pass through the French *jeu d'espirit* in order to rediscover Freud's discovery—that symptoms are ways of speaking and, like all communications, only take meaning in a specific context.[2] Just as Cixous's Dora refuses the substitutability of all women, psychoanalysis (and feminism) must refuse the substitutability of all cases, the "well-known sort of key" ("It is *well known* what sort of 'key' effects the opening in such a *case*").

It is not just the English translator who puts the Dora text through French detours; Freud himself interjected French phrases at certain points in his German text. The most remarkable one, one that Cixous writes into her play (p. 36), is the sentence "J'appelle un chat un chat" (literally, "I call a cat a cat"; compare the English "call a spade a spade"). The context is once again the question of scandal, here specifically that the reader might be scandalized that a psychoanalyst should discuss sexual practices, especially perverse sexual practices (in this case, oral intercourse) with an inexperienced girl.

Freud writes, "A gynaecologist, after all, under the same conditions, does not hesitate to *make them submit to uncovering every possible part of their body*. The *best way* of speaking about such things *is to be dry and direct*" (my italics). Freud concludes his argument thus: "I call bodily organs and processes by their technical names, and I tell these to the patient if they—the names, I mean—happen to be unknown to her. *J'appelle un chat un chat*" (*SE* 7:48; *C* 65). At the very moment he defines nonprurient language as direct and noneuphemistic, he takes a French detour into a figurative expression. By his terms, this French sentence would seem to be titillating, coy, flirtatious. And to make matters more juicy (less "dry"), *chat* or *chatte* can be used as vulgar (vulvar) slang for the female genitalia. So in this gynecological context, where he founds his innocence upon the direct use of technical terms, he takes a French detour and calls a pussy a pussy.[3]

Freud's defensive interjection, "the names, I mean," leads us back to a passage where he writes that he "took the greatest pains with this patient not to introduce her to any fresh facts in the region of sexual knowledge. . . . I did not call a thing by its name until her allusions to it had become so unambiguous that there seemed slight risk in translating them into direct speech." (SE 7:31; *C* 46). Freud restricts his activities to translation from allusive to "direct speech." But as we have seen, "direct speech" leads to "j'appelle un chat un chat," that is, translation from German into French, from scientific into figurative language, from original expression into cliché. The innocent activity Freud calls "translation" seems to relate to some kind of suspicious *détour* that allows repression to be evaded.

The passage continues: "Her answer was always prompt and frank: she knew about it already. But the question of where her knowledge came from was a riddle which her memories were unable to solve." Freud is *not* the author of her knowledge (merely the translator), but who is? As translator of an anonymous text, his responsibility (or lack of it) is more ambiguous. The "riddle" is not solved until it is too late, until a footnote to the Postface, where Freud writes, "I *ought to have* guessed that the main source of her knowledge of sexual matters could have been no one but Frau K. . . . I *ought to have* attacked this riddle and looked for the motive of *such an extraordinary piece of repression*" (*SE* 7:120 *n.; C* 142 *n.;* my italics). Why did Freud fail to do what he "ought to have"? Why did he not attack the riddle?

In *Portrait de Dora,* Freud's line "*J'appelle un chat un chat*" is spoken by Frau K. (p. 36). This sets up an identification between the "author" of Dora's sexual knowledge and its "translator." Is Freud afraid of solving the riddle because, like Oedipus, he will find himself to be the guilty party?

In a way, yes. But not because of any direct identification with Frau K. Before he finally solves the riddle, Freud arrives at a preliminary solution. "For some time," Freud writes in a footnote, "I looked upon [Dora's governess] as the source of all Dora's secret knowledge, and perhaps I was not entirely wrong in this" *(SE* 7:36 *n.; C* 52*n.).* It is precisely in the position of the governess, of the servant, that Dora places Freud.

When Dora announces that they are in their last session, Freud asks her when she decided to terminate the analysis. To her response, "a fortnight ago," Freud replies, "That sounds just like a maidservant or a governess—a fortnight's warning." Is the servant giving two weeks' notice before quitting, or is the master giving the servant two weeks' notice before letting her go? In other words, is Dora or Freud in the role of the governess? Cixous's play gives a double reading to this, leaving the distribution of roles ambiguous. In the play, Freud says: "A fortnight? That's the notice a governess gives of her departure" (p. 98). In this reading the departing one, Dora, is the governess. But, in response to Dora's complaint that the cure is lasting too long, Freud says: "You still need a helper for several months"; Dora replies, "I don't need a governess" (p. 82). Perhaps the only respect in which this ambiguity can be decided is economic. Freud is being paid by Dora's family; he is the servant whose services are no longer required. I certainly do not wish to deny the Dora-governess identification, but merely to emphasize what is *not* analyzed in Freud's text.

As Cixous points out, there are two governesses in Dora's story, and both suffer the same fate—seduced and abandoned by the master (*La jeune née,* p. 276). When Freud makes the governess connection in

Dora's last session, she recalls the K.'s governess, who had been seduced by Herr K. with the same words he then tried to use on Dora. When Dora transfers her relation to Herr K. onto Freud, she refuses to be dismissed as the governess was. Her revenge is to switch roles and put Herr K./Freud into the place of the servant and dismiss him.

The identification between Freud and the governess does not result merely from Dora's revenge reversal. Dora told how *her* governess appeared to be interested in Dora until Dora realized the governess was really just interested in Dora's father (*SE* 7:37; *C* 53). Octave Mannoni, in his *Fictions freudiennes,* has Dora write a letter to Frau K. in which she says that Freud, likewise, "was not really interested in me, but only in pleasing papa" (p. 15). If it is the case that Freud is using Dora to get to her father—that, as Mannoni has Dora say, Freud is "in love with papa" (p. 15)–then it is ironic that Freud should suffer the same fate as the governess, to be rejected by Dora's father. Freud writes at the end of the case history,

> *It must be confessed* that Dora's father was *never entirely straightforward.* He had *given his support* to the treatment so long as he could hope that I should "talk" Dora out of her belief that there was something more than a friendship between him and Frau K. *His interest faded* when he observed that it was not my intention to bring about that result." (*SE* 7:109; C 131; my italics)

"It must be confessed" suggests that there is some shame attached to this for Freud. He has been taken in, believing in this man's "interest" and "support," and then discovering he was merely being used.

Identification between Freud and a governess, maid, or nurse is not restricted to the confines of the Dora case but has a decisive, structural relation to psychoanalysis in general. Psychoanalysis—Freud was discovering at the time of the Dora case but not "in time"—works because of the transference, because the patient transfers previous relations with others onto the psychoanalyst, reactivates the emotions, and can work them out in analysis. Later Freud will theorize that all relations to others merely repeat the child's original relation to the mother, the first other. Transference is not peculiar to psychoanalysis but is actually the structure of all love. Even the relation to the father, Freud discovered, is already actually a transference of mother-love onto the father. What distinguishes psychoanalysis from other relations is the possibility of analyzing the transference, of being aware of the emotions as a repetition, as inappropriate to context. Whereas in other relationships both parties have an investment in seeing love not as a repetition but as unique and particular to the person loved, in psychoanalysis the analyst will want to point out the structure of repetition. What facilitates the recognition of the feeling as transference, as an inappropriate repetition, is the fact that the analyst is paid. The money proves that the analyst is only a stand-in. Rather than having the power of life and death like the mother has over the infant, the analyst is financially dependent on the patient. But, in that case, the original "analyst," the earliest person paid to replace the mother, is that frequent character in Freud's histories, the nursemaid/governess.

And she is, as both Clément and Cixous agreed, the ultimate seductress (p. 276). Just as the Dora case poses for Freud the "riddle" of the source of Dora's sexual knowledge, hysteria in general poses the enigma of a seduction, that is, likewise, an initiation into carnal knowledge. In the first section of *La jeune née* ("La Coupable"—The Guilty Woman), Clément traces Freud's search for the guilty one, his search for the seducer. Freud begins with the discovery that hysterics were seduced by their fathers. But unable to accept the possibility of so many perverse fathers, he presses on to the discovery of infantile, polymorphous perverse sexuality. Not fathers but children are perverse: they fantasize seduction by the father. But his detective work does not stop there. Perhaps because he is a father and was a child, he goes on to locate the guilt where it will not besmirch him. He will escape Oedipus' fate, and his search for the original sin will end up exculpating him as father/child. In the 1933 lecture "Femininity" he writes: "And now we find the phantasy of seduction once more in the pre-Oedipus . . . but the seducer is regularly the mother. Here, however, the phantasy touches the ground of reality, for it was really the mother who by her activities over the child's bodily hygiene inevitably stimulated, and perhaps even roused for the first time, pleasurable sensations in her genitals" (*SE* 22:120). Whereas the fantasy of the father's seduction is mere fantasy, the mother's seduction "touches the ground of reality." This "ground of reality," the mother's actual role in child raising, assures that there is no realistic ground for identification between Freud and the mother. The riddle is solved: the mother is "the source" of sexuality, of perversion, of neurosis. The detective work is completed.

Or it would be completed if the family were truly a closed circuit. One of psychoanalysis's consistent errors is to reduce everything to a family paradigm. Sociopolitical questions are always brought back to the model father–mother–child. Class conflict and revolution are understood as a repetition of parent–child relations. This has always been the pernicious apoliticism of psychoanalysis. It has also been hard to argue against without totally rejecting psychoanalysis, since it is based upon the fundamental notion that everything we do as adults must repeat some infantile wish, and for most of us, the infantile world was the family. What is necessary to get beyond this dilemma is a recognition that the closed, cellular model of the family used in such psychoanalytic thinking is an idealization, a secondary revision of the family. The family never was, in any of Freud's texts, completely closed off from questions of economic class. And the most insistent locus of that intrusion into the family circle (intrusion of the symbolic into the imaginary) is the maid/governess/nurse. As Cixous says, "She is the hole in the social cell."[4]

The search for the seducer is not complete when it has interrogated all the family members: father–child–mother. "Femininity," the text quoted earlier, in which Freud declares the mother's seduction as grounded in reality, might be considered a secondary revision of an earlier text, "Female Sexuality." In this earlier text we read: "The part played in starting [phallic activity] by nursery hygiene is reflected in the very common phantasy which makes the mother or nurse into a seducer. . . . Actual seduction, too, is common enough; it is initiated either by other children or someone in charge of the child [nursemaid]—who wants to soothe it, or send it to sleep or make it dependent on them" (*SE* 21:232).

It has become a commonplace of the history of psychoanalysis to mark as a turning point the moment in the 1890s when Freud stopped believing in a "real" seduction at the origin of hysteria and realized that the source of neurosis is the child's fantasies. This is the monumental break with theories of traumatic etiology and the discovery of infantile sexuality. But here, in a 1931 text, Freud is talking about "actual seduction." The father cannot be a seducer; that would undercut his upright position as patriarch. Even the mother only seduces unwittingly in the execution of her proper duties. The "actual seduction," intentional seduction, can only be the act of another child (children, not parents, are perverse) or a nurse. The servant, member of a lower class, like a child, is capable of perversion.

The discovery of the universal fantasy of seduction by the father is Freud's discovery of the Oedipus complex. From that, via *Totem and Taboo,* we reach an incest taboo that, formulated by Lévi-Strauss, will found society by keeping sexual relations outside the family circle. If sexual relations are understood as some kind of contact with alterity (although generally there is some ritual homogenization of that alterity), then the incest taboo would institute a prohibition against alterity within the family circle, a law ensuring the "imaginary" closure of the cell. In that case, the "nurse"—not only outside the family but outside the economic class—would constitute the greatest threat to the law homogenizing the family. Lévi-Strauss finds that the correlate to the incest taboo is endogamy. Sexual relations are with someone whose alterity is limited within the confines of a larger circle. Exogamy, marrying outside the larger circle, is equally a violation of the incest taboo. Marriage outside of class or race might represent a contact with a nonassimilable alterity, thus like actual incest bringing unmitigated heterogeneity within the family circle. Freud's nurses and governesses might represent just such otherness, the very otherness that can also be represented by the violence of class conflict. Yet she is there at the heart of the family, in the cell nucleus. She is so much part of the family that the child's fantasies (the unconscious) do not distinguish "mother or nurse."

The question Clément asked about the hysteric must be asked about the governess. Does she contest or conserve? Is she a heroine or a victim? Is she a hole in the cell (as Cixous says), or does the cell close up around her again? "Open" or "shut" cannot be a matter of indifference. Of course, the answer is that her role is ambiguous. ("I was 'sure' you would say that.") The determining question is one of symbolic inscription. The apolitical psychoanalytic thinking that has traditionally reduced economic questions to "family matters" is simply an avatar of familial thinking. The familial imaginary wants to preserve the infantile fantasmatic confusion between mother and nurse. If the nurse is assimilated to the mother (if the transference goes unquestioned), then the family cell can close up again.

Psychoanalysis can and ought to be the place of symbolic inscription of the governess. The absolute importance of the economic transaction between patient and analyst has been repeatedly stressed by analytic theory. Despite this, there is a strong temptation to be the Mother (the phallic mother, Lacan's Other, the subject presumed to know, the Doctor) rather than the nurse. Freud, for example, used to raise money to support the Wolf Man, after the latter was impoverished. The Wolf Man is the classic case of a patient who never resolved the transference, who remained "Freud's Wolf Man" for the rest of his life. How can the transference be analyzed if the economic rupture of the imaginary is sutured, the financial distinction between governess and mother effaced? For psychoanalysis to be a locus of radical contestation, Freud must assume his identification with the governess.

Cixous says in *La jeune née,* "The truth is that, in the system of exchange, me in your place and you in my place, . . . Freud in relation to Dora occupied the maid's place. It is Freud who was the maid, and that is what is intolerable for Freud in the Dora case, it's to have been treated like maids are treated: to have been thrown out like maids were thrown out" (p. 280). The vulgar, idiomatic expression Cixous uses for "thrown out" is *"foutu à la porte." Foutre,* which no longer has a literal sense, used to mean "fuck." What Freud could not tolerate was to "have been *foutu à la porte* (fucked at the door) like maids were fucked at the door." I take leave for this vulgar, literal reading from Cixous's emphasis on the door feature in Dora *(Porte–trait de Door-a),* which keeps the door in this commonplace idiom from facing into a figurative background. Once the door is noticed, *"foutre"* is unavoidable. The maid is "fucked at the door." She is "at the door" inasmuch as she is a threshold figure: existing between "within the family" and "outside the family." Fucking her is a threshold act, somewhere between incest and exogamy, participating in both, embracing the outside, all the while attempting to assimilate it. If "open" or "shut" is not a matter of indifference, as Freud would have it, then *"foutre"* always takes place "at the door." It is not just the maid, but in Freud's "well-known" symbolism, women in general who are *"foutues à la porte."*

As Cixous points out, the Dora case is punctuated by women being declared "nothing" (*La jeune née,* p. 281). Both Herr K. and Dora's father say that of their wives.[5] What is true of the wives (mothers) is even more explicit for the two governesses. Dora "sees a massacre of women executed to make space for her. But she knows that she will in turn be massacred" (p. 282). Neither Dora, the hysteric, nor Freud, the governess, can tolerate the position allotted them by the system of exchanges. Neither Dora nor Freud can tolerate identification with the seduced and abandoned governess.

As a threatening representative of the symbolic, the economic, the extrafamilial, the maid must be both seduced (assimilated) and abandoned (expelled). She must be *"foutue à la porte."* The nurse is desirable; her alterity is a stimulus, a tension, a disturbing itch in the composure of the family. But the desire for her is murderous. Sexual seduction (ritual homogenizing assimilation) is not sufficient to reduce the stimulus tension. Her alterity is not just her femininity, not even just her not belonging to the family, it is her not belonging to the same economic class. It is not enough to seduce her; she must be expelled from the family.

Dora and Freud cannot bear to identify with the governess because they think there is still some place where one can escape the structural exchange of women. They still believe that there is some mother who is not a governess. Both Dora and Freud dismiss Dora's mother; she is obviously not the phallic mother. But Dora refuses to blame or resent Frau K., refuses to see the similarity between Frau K. and the governess, who was using Dora to please Dora's father. Her love for Frau K.—the adoration of her that is brought out by Cixous's play, as well as Lacan's reading of the Dora case[6]—is a belief in her phallic uniqueness, her nonsubstitutability. That she should be compared to the Madonna (by Lacan and Cixous) is instructive in this regard.

Freud's and Dora's understanding of the "barter" of women never passes through the general term "des femmes," always remains in the imaginary. The imaginary might be characterized as the realm of nonassumption of the mother's castration. In the imaginary, the "mother," unlike the maid, is assumed to be still phallic; omnipotent and omniscient, she is unique. What shows in the Dora case that neither Dora nor Freud wanted to see is that Frau K. and Dora's mother are in the same position as the maid. In feminist or symbolic or economic terms the mother/wife is in a position of substitutability and economic inferiority. For the analysis to pass out of the imaginary, it must pass through a symbolic third term—like "des femmes" on the cover of Cixous's *Portrait de Dora,* a term that represents a class.

Having reached a definite conclusion, I find more remains to be said. The "more" revolves around Dora's love for Frau K., around her lesbianism. This supplementary postscript would repeat Freud's gesture of emphasizing Dora's homosexual love in a footnote to his conclusion.

What has been said of that love in the present text is that Dora sees Frau K. as the phallic mother, infallible, nonsubstitutable. My argument has subordinated this homosexual love to the important psychoanalytic and feminist question of the relation between transference and radical contestation. Dora's love for Frau K. has been cited here as an instance of the imaginary, which is to be taken as a criticism. But the "more" I have to say is about the beauty, the eroticism, the affirmative quality of that love, a side brought out particularly by Cixous's *Portrait.* And somehow beauty and affirmation, sexuality as pleasure and joy rather than as murderous assimilation, seem to find their place only as a supplement to the political, theoretical argument.

This afterthought also repeats a gesture Cixous makes in the dialogue at the end of *La jeune née.* She says that Dora "saw the ignominy and the staging of the murder of woman. *One should add to that* what there is in Dora of a very beautiful, staggering, feminine homosexuality, what there is of love of woman" (p. 282; my italics). The first sentence quoted here is the climax of Cixous's argument that Dora saw and refused the "massacre" involved in the "barter" of woman. This is the political analysis that constitutes Cixous' reading of the Dora case. But rather than conclude there, Cixous feels the need of something more, so she continues mid-paragraph: "One should add to that." Perhaps in a theoretical text one can never do more than say "There is more, there is love and beauty," which is a necessary affirmative supplement to the murderous negation that theory must be. But in *Portrait de Dora*, in the theatrical text, in the fiction, this is not a problem; the affirmative is interwoven in various patterns with the negative.[7]

The argument I conclude above, before this postscript, accepts Clément's valuation of symbolic inscription. The symbolic is politically healthy; the imaginary is regressive. That is a classic Lacanian ethical hierarchy. But like all hierarchies, it can be oppressive. One of the effects of this hierarchy, of all hierarchies (Cixous suggests, pp. 115–117), is to support the valuation of men over women. The symbolic is linked to the Law of the Father, to the Phallus, whereas the imaginary is linked to the relation to the Mother. There have been some thinkers who have questioned this valuation of the symbolic at the expense of the imaginary. Two of the most eloquent in their questioning are Jean Laplanche and Michèle Montrelay.[8] Both argue that Lacanian analysts have been so preoccupied with denouncing the ego and thus the imaginary (for the ego is the agency of the imaginary), that they have overlooked the positive and necessary function of the imaginary. Lacanian theory views the imaginary as a "pure effect of the symbolic," but it might also be said that the imaginary is necessary to give "consistency" to the symbolic (Montrelay), to "embody" it (Laplanche). Since the imaginary embodies, fleshes out the skeletal symbolic, it is possible to see the Lacanian devaluation of the imaginary as related to a hatred of the flesh, of woman and of pleasure.

Clément denies her love for the hysterics—"I really liked them, but they no longer exist"—whereas she accuses Cixous of really liking Dora. Clément has passed into the symbolic and wants to keep this love safely behind her, in the past tense, does not want to regress into the imaginary. Dora's love for Frau K. is marked in Freud's text by Dora's phrase "her adorable white body" (p. 61). In Cixous's play Dora describes this body as "pearly" (p. 34). Yet Clément, in her section of *La jeune née*, calls Dora "the pearl of the hysterics" (p. 96). It is not that Clément does not love Dora but that she wants to deny that love, the beauty of the pearl, wants to be firmly ensconced in the symbolic, with no ambiguity.

It cannot be a question here of choosing Clément's symbolic or Cixous's imaginary. Indeed, the fact that the two are bound together into one book frustrates traditional notions of opposition. Like the hysteric's role, like the governess's role, we must learn to accept the ambiguity, learn to make "open or shut" a matter of indifference. Both Clément and Cixous use the word "bisexual" in their texts in *La jeune née* to name some sort of positive goal. Bisexuality has traditionally been linked with hysteria in psychoanalytic theory. But these women writers are talking about an "other bisexuality." Neither the fantasmatic resolution of differences in the imaginary, nor the fleshless, joyless assumption of the fact of one's lack of unity in the symbolic, but an other bisexuality, one that pursues, loves, and accepts both the imaginary and the symbolic, both theory and flesh.

Notes

1. Catherine Clément and Hélène Cixous, *La jeune née* (Paris: 10/18, 1975), p. 184.

2. There is one other example in the Dora case where the English translation uses a French phrase to render Freud's German: "And if the connection between the symptomatic expression and the unconscious mental content should strike us as being in this case a clever *tour de force,* we shall be glad to hear it succeeds in creating the same impression in every other case and in every other instance." Again what Freud is discussing here is the scandalous discovery that the unconscious speaks. The French work which insists on his discovery might be suspected by Anglophones as a "clever *tour de force,*" that is artful and far-fetched rather than serious and scientific.

3. In the next paragraph Freud uses another French expression—*pour faire une omelette il faut casser des oeufs* (you have to break eggs to make an omelette)—still in the context of his defense of sexual conversation with his hysterics. Yet even this culinary commonplace can take on a sexual meaning. Lacan, in "Position de l'inconscient" (*Écrits),* rewrites "omelette" into its near homonym "hommelette"—homunculus or little man. One could, following that lead, read the proverb as meaning "you have to break eggs (penetrate and fertilize ova) to make a little man (a baby)."

4. *La jeune née,* p. 276. There is a nurse in Freud's own infancy who plays an important role and is connected to "cases" and being "locked up." She was expelled from the house and locked up for theft. See Ernest Jones, *Sigmund Freud: Life and Work,* vol. 1 (New York: Basic Books, 1953). For some excellent work on the import of Freud's nurse, see Jim Swan, "*Mater* and Nannie," *American Imago* (Spring 1974), vol. 31, no. 1.

5. Actually, in the English translation they say, "I get nothing out of my wife," whereas Cixous has them say in French, "My wife is nothing for me." Probably the most literal translation of the German—*Ich habe nichts an meiner Frau*—would be, "I have nothing in my wife." What seems to work, regardless of the language, is an insistent association between "wife" and "nothing."

6. See Lacan's excellent and unusually clear "Intervention sur le transfert," in *Ecrits* (essay 4 in this book).

7. But must we accept this inevitable division? Cannot a theoretical text also be theatrical? "Theatre" and "theory" both stem from the same root—"thea." In fact, is theory not always theatrical, a rhetorical performance as well as a quest for truth? The limits of theory remain to be tested.

8. Michèle Montrelay, *L'ombre et le nom*, (Paris: Editions de Minuit, 1977), pp. 155–156. Jean Laplanche, *Life and Death in Psychoanalysis*, Jeffrey Mehlman, tr. (Baltimore: Johns Hopkins University Press, 1976), pp. 125–126.

10. Dora's Secrets, Freud's Techniques

NEIL HERTZ

WHAT DORA KNEW

Imagine an older man intrigued by the following story: a young girl is drawn—perhaps in all innocence, perhaps in frightened or even fascinated complicity—into an adult, adulterous sexual tangle involving her father and an Other Woman, a woman she had come to trust. How would this play itself out, how would the daughter's observations and principles make themselves felt? How would she bear the burden of her knowledge? What would that knowledge do to her? Add to this set of questions another set, of equal interest to the older man: How can this story be told? Who can tell it? Can the daughter tell it unaided? Or must her account be supplemented and revised by a more informed, a more articulate, adult consciousness? And if it is so supplemented, how can the adult be sure he is getting the story straight, setting it down in unadulterated form? That is, how can he be sure that his telling of the story isn't itself a further violation of the young girl's particular integrity?

I have been paraphrasing bits of Henry James' Preface to *What Maisie*

This article was first published in *Diacritics* (Spring 1983), pp. 65–76.

Knew, but paraphrasing rather selectively, blurring the considerable differences between Maisie's story and Dora's so as to dwell on the ways the two stories, and the concerns of their authors, overlap. James and Freud alike anticipate being reproached for both the nature of the stories they have to tell and for the manner of the telling. And both meet these imagined reproaches in ways that suggest that the two faults might be one, that they run the risk of being accused of a perverse and distasteful confusion, of not striking the right balance between the child's world and the adult's. There is, to begin with, the possibility that each is gratuitously dragging his heroine into more knowledge, more sordid knowledge, than girls of her age need to come to terms with. Here is James:

> Of course . . . I was punctually to have had read to me the lesson that the "mixing-up" of a child with anything unpleasant confessed itself an aggravation of the unpleasantness, and that nothing could well be more disgusting than to attribute to Maisie so intimate an "acquaintance" with the gross immoralities surrounding her.[1]

and Freud, answering a similar charge:

> There is never any danger of corrupting an inexperienced girl. For where there is no knowledge of sexual processes even in the unconscious, no hysterical symptom will arise; and where hysteria is found there can no longer be any question of "innocence of mind" in the sense in which parents and educators use the phrase. (SE 7:49; *C* 66)

Furthermore, there is the possibility that both authors are (in dangerous and, it is hinted, somehow self-serving ways) imposing not experience but language on the less sophisticated consciousness of the child. Freud meets the charge with a familiar distinction: "With the exercise of a little caution all that is done is to translate into conscious ideas what was already known in the unconscious" (*SE* 7:49; *C* 66). James, too, imagines himself chiefly as his heroine's interpreter and, like Freud, assumes that there is some fund of knowledge there not immediately accessible but peculiarly worth the effort of translation:

> Small children have many more perceptions then they have terms to translate them; their vision is at any moment much richer, their apprehension even

constantly stronger, than their prompt, their at all producible vocabulary. Amusing therefore as it might at the first blush have seemed to restrict myself in this case to the terms as well as to the experience, it became at once plain that such an attempt would fail. Maisie's terms accordingly play their part—since her simpler conclusions quite depend on them; but our own commentary constantly attends and amplifies. This it is that on occasion, doubtless, seems to represent us as going so "behind" the facts of her spectacle as to exaggerate the activity of her relation to them. The difference here is but of a shade: it is her relation, her activity of spirit, that determines all our own concern—we simply take advantage of these things better than she herself. Only, even though it is her interest that mainly makes matters interesting for us, we inevitably note this in figures that are not yet at her command and that are nevertheless required whenever those aspects about her and those parts of her experience that she understands darken off into others that she rather tormentedly misses. (p. 146)

Just here our analogy may begin to show signs of strain, however. Freud is writing about translating "what was already known in the unconscious" of a young patient whose mind was by no means an open book; James, on the other, is Maisie's creator: how can he pretend that anything impedes his knowing the contents of her mind? We may think we know what he means: Maisie may be a fiction, but children are real, and relatively opaque to adult inspection. Some distance is inevitable, some interpretative effort required. But as James goes on to write of Maisie, in sentences which exhibit that odd dexterity that allows a novelist to speak of his characters almost in the same breath both as products of his imagination and as autonomous beings, we sense that James' interest in Maisie is not simply that of a mimetic artist challenging himself to produce a tour de force of accuracy. The note of admiration we catch in the Preface suggests that, whatever it is that Maisie knew, James envies that knowledge and sets a peculiarly high value on it. His own language darkens with hints of mourning, then glows in intense pastoral identification, when he speaks of her:

Successfully to resist (to resist, that is, the strain of observation and the assault of experience) what would that be, on the part of so young a person, but to remain fresh, and still fresh, and to have even a freshness to communicate?—the case being with Maisie to the end that she treats her friends to the rich little spectacle of objects embalmed in her wonder. She wonders, in other words, to the end, to the death—the death of her childhood, properly speaking; . . . She is not only the extraordinary "ironic centre" I have already noted; she has the wonderful importance of shedding a light far beyond any reach of her comprehension; of lending to poorer persons and things, by the mere fact of their being involved with her and by the special scale she creates for them, a precious element of dignity. I lose myself, truly, in appreciation of my theme on noting what she does by her "freshness" for appearances in themselves vulgar and empty enough. They become, as she deals with them, the stuff of poetry and tragedy and art; she has simply to wonder, as I say, about them, and they begin to have meanings, aspects, solidities, connexions—connexions with the "universal!"—that they could scarce have hoped for. (p. 147)

Maisie's "wonder"—and this seems to be its value for James—both illuminates and embalms; she, in turn, remains fresh and yet wonders "to the end, to the death—the death of her childhood." Although the novel concludes with Maisie alive, having weathered "the assault of experience," this strong but fleeting touch of pathos nevertheless suggests a thematics of sacrifice and compensation. The figurative death Maisie is said to endure is made to seem the price paid for the remarkable transforming effects of her wonder, her embalming of what is inherently "vulgar and empty enough" into "the stuff of poetry," that is, into the matter of the novel. *What Maisie Knew,* James seems to be claiming, could not have been written if he hadn't had access to what Maisie in fact knew, and it is she who—at some large but indeterminate cost to herself—somehow made that possible. "I lose myself, truly, in appreciation of my theme on noting what she does by her 'freshness' ": the shifting personal pronouns trace the distribution of fond investment here—it is simultaneously beamed at "myself," at "my theme," and at "her." Nor is it clear where one of these agents or sources of value and power leaves off and another begins: James is writing out of a strong identification with a composite idea/theme/character/surrogate/muse. When he speaks of the death of Maisie's childhood, we can take that phrase as gesturing toward her growing up (and out of the world of this particular story) but also as figuring the collapse of that charged distance and equivocal commerce between James and his surrogate that attends the completion of the novel.

We are accustomed to these modes of imaginative identification—and to the confusions they give rise to—in considering the genesis of works of fiction; when we turn to the relation of a psychoanalyst to his patient, or of the author of a case history to its central character, we are more prepared to believe that the forms of fantasmatic confusion we are likely to encounter are classifiable as transferential or countertransferential effects. And, indeed, much of the reconsideration of Freud's dealing with Dora—as her therapist and as the teller of her story—has tended to appraise his work in these terms. If Freud, as he himself acknowledged, failed to heal Dora, or if his account of her, what Philip Rieff refers to as his "brilliant yet barbaric" account of her,[2] failed to get at the truth of her case, it is usually held to be because he did not notice, or did not give sufficient weight to, the ways in which Dora was burdening him with feelings about her father, or Herr K., or the governess, or Frau K.; or he was insufficiently alert to his own erotic or paternal or erotico-paternal feelings about Dora; or—to extend this allusion to the counter-transference into a sociological or historical dimension—Freud's attitudes toward young, unmarried, unhappy women shared the blindness and exploitative bent of the prevailing patriarchal culture. Each of these accusations can be made to stick; I shall be taking them for granted and pursuing another line of questioning.

Suppose what went wrong between Freud and Dora was not just a matter of unrecognized transferences (and countertransferences) but also of an unrecognized—or refused—identification? Suppose what Freud missed, or did not wish to see, was not that he was drawn to (or repelled by) Dora, but that he "was" Dora, or rather that the question of who was who was more radically confusing than even nuanced accounts of unacknowledged transferences and countertransferences suggest? Is it possible that one of the sources of energy and of distortion in the "Fragment of an Analaysis" is to be located here, in the confusion of tongues between an author and his young surrogate, and that we can find in Freud's text some of the extravagant tones as well as some of the gestures of sacrifice and self-location that inform James' writing about Maisie? We can find them, I believe, but with this telling difference: that the kind of fancied identification that can be happily, even amusedly acknowledged by James will represent something more of a threat to Freud. The "Fragment of an Analysis" exhibits the grounds for such a confusion and the means by which Freud fended it off.

RETICENCE

A first point of resemblance: neither Dora nor Freud tells all. In Dora's case it would seem to be because she simply cannot: how could she either reveal or intentionally conceal secrets she does not know she has? As for Freud, he would seem to be consciously—but not willfully—choosing what he will communicate to his readers:

> There is another kind of incompleteness which I myself have intentionally introduced. I have as a rule not reproduced the process of interpretation to which the patient's associations and communications had to be subjected, but only the results of that process. Apart from the dreams, therefore, the technique of the analytic work has been revealed in only a very few places. My object in this case history was to demonstrate the intimate structure of a neurotic disorder and the determination of its symptoms; and it would have led to nothing but hopeless confusion if I had tried to complete the other task at the same time. (*SE* 7:12–13; *C* 27)

This decision not to say much about "the technique of the analytic work," or what he calls elsewhere in the text—and repeatedly until the word *technique* and its cognates come to seem peculiarly salient—"psychoanalytic technique," "the technical rules," "the technical work," etc., hardly qualifies as a concealment, once the reasons for such prudence have been so sensibly set forth. Yet as the case history goes on, Freud renews his reminders of what it is he will not talk about, and often in contexts that lend them a puzzling resonance. Here, for example, he is discussing the relation between unconscious sexual fantasies and the production of hysterical symptoms:

> An opportunity very soon occurred for interpreting Dora's nervous cough in this way by means of an imagined sexual situation. She had once again been insisting that Frau K. only loved her father because he was "*ein vermögender*

Mann" [a man of means]. Certain details of the way in which she expressed herself (which I pass over here, like most other purely technical parts of the analysis) led me to see that behind this phrase its opposite lay concealed, namely, that her father was "*ein unvermögender Man*" [a man without means]. This could only be meant in a sexual sense—that her father, as a man, was without means, was impotent. Dora confirmed this interpretation from her conscious knowledge; whereupon I pointed out the contradiction she was involved in if on the one hand she continued to insist that her father's relation with Frau K. was a common love-affair, and on the other hand maintained that her father was impotent, or in other words incapable of carrying on an affair of such a kind. Her answer showed that she had no need to admit the contradiction. She knew very well, she said, that there was more than one way of obtaining sexual gratification. (The source of this piece of knowledge, however, was once more untraceable.) I questioned her further, whether she referred to the use of organs other than the genitals for the purpose of sexual intercourse, and she replied in the affirmative. (SE 7:47; *C* 64)

It is the question of knowledge that makes possible comparisons between doctor and patient here. For the relation between them is not as assymmetrical as it might be if Dora were suffering from some organic disease. If that were the case, Freud's techniques would be diagnostic procedures of one sort or another and would in no way resemble Dora's as yet unknown and hence "secret" condition. But Dora's condition is, in fact, her way of living *her* knowledge: a number of secrets lie behind her symptoms, some easier for Freud to get at than others, but all turning on what Dora knew. There is what she can confirm "from her conscious knowledge"—her awareness of male impotence, her knowing "very well" that there are various paths to sexual gratification—as well as secrets more elusive, the "source" of what she knew, for example. Or the relation between what she knows and what she suffers, the complicated set of mediations, fantasmatic and physiological, which Freud characterizes as "the intimate structure of a neurotic disorder" (*SE* 7:13; *C* 27) or "the finer structure of a neurosis" (*SE* 7:12; *C* 26) or "the internal structure of her hysteria" (*SE* 7:112, *C* 134). It is in the course of pursuing these connections and uncovering that intimate structure that a further point of resemblance between Freud and his patient becomes noticeable. To pick up where the previous citation left off:

> . . . she replied in the affirmative. I could then go on to say that in that case she must be thinking of precisely those parts of the body which in her case were in a state of irritation—the throat and the oral cavity. To be sure, she would not hear of going so far as this in recognizing her own thoughts; and indeed, if the occurrence of the symptom was to be made possible at all, it was essential that she should not be completely clear on the subject. But the conclusion was inevitable that with her spasmodic cough, which, as is usual, was referred for its exciting cause to a tickling in her throat, she pictured to herself a scene of sexual gratification *per os* between the two people whose love-affair occupied her mind so incessantly. A very short time after she had tacitly accepted this explanation her cough vanished—which fitted in very well with my view. (*SE* 7:47–8; *C* 64–65)

Dora's lack of clarity on the relation between her cough and her father's affair is captured in the slight abstraction of the language in which the sexual scenario is presented: "she pictured herself a scene of sexual gratification *per os.*" As in the fantasy Freud called "A Child Is Being Beaten," in which the fantast can occupy any of three positions—that of the child, that of the person punishing him, or that of an excited onlooker—it is not clear from this sentence who is gratifying whom, *per* whose *os* the pleasure is being procured, or with whom Dora is identifying. But it is not clear, either, just who is not being clear here, Dora or Freud. Freud certainly intends to be clear: he will go on to refer to the sexual act as one in which a woman is "sucking at the male organ" (*SE* 7:51; *C* 68); he seems convinced that what Dora knows about is fellatio. But that isn't immediately obvious: in Jacques Lacan's commentary on the case he remarks, very much in passing, in the course of correcting Freud on Dora's relation to Frau K. and to femininity in general, that, of course, "everyone knows that cunnilingus is the artifice most commonly adopted by 'men of means' whose powers begin to abandon them" (see essay 4). It is hard to guess what Freud would have made of this note of high Parisian *savoir vivre;* whatever everyone else knew, he seems to have taken for granted the more phallic—and phallocentric—option.

But if this is, as Freud's feminist critics have pointed out, a stereotypical prejudice, it is also compact with some other factors in Freud's thinking that engage questions of oral intercourse in the other sense of that term. He next turns, in what appears to be a slight digression but is nonetheless thematically continuous with the previous discussion, to anticipate the "astonishment and horror" a hypothetical "medical reader" may feel on learning that Freud dares "talk about such delicate and unpleasant subjects to a young girl" or that there is a possibility that an "inexperienced girl could know about practices of such a kind and could occupy her imagination with them" (*SE* 7:48; *C* 65). There are those, he goes on, "who are scandalized by a therapeutic method in which conversations of this sort occur, and who appear to envy either me or my patients the titillation which, according to their notions, such a method must afford." Earlier, he had anticipated the same objection—specifically that psychoanalytic conversation is "a good means of exciting or gratifying sexual desires" (*SE* 7:9; *C* 23), and he had defended himself, as he does here, by insisting that his practice is no more gratifying in this respect than that of a gynecologist. What is thrust aside is the possibility of the doctor's deriving pleasure from these oral exchanges: it is the gynecologist's willed professional anesthesia that is being invoked here:

> The best way of speaking about such things is to be dry and direct; and that is at the same time the method furthest removed from the prurience with which the same subjects are handled in "society," and to which girls and women alike are so thoroughly accustomed. I call bodily organs and processes by their technical names, and I tell these to the patient if they—the names, I mean—happen to be unknown to her. (*SE* 7:48; *C* 65)

"Technical" here means, among other things, "unexciting": and if this explanation of Freud's is both honest and convincing, it also has the (unintended) result of aligning his own refusal-of-pleasure with the "internal structure" he has just been describing at work in Dora, the repressive mechanism whereby a distinctly uncomfortable symptom had been substituted for a possibly pleasurable voyeuristic fantasy. Dora refuses to "know" that when she coughs she is picturing to herself a scene of oral gratification; and Freud has every reason to deny that his own conversations with girls like Dora are titillating. What she secretly represses he subdues through a consciously elaborated professional technique.[3]

SOURCES OF KNOWLEDGE

A psychoanalyst can resemble his patient in eschewing sexual pleasure; on her side, a patient can resemble her psychoanalyst in the intensity with which she pursues secret knowledge—or so, at least, the language of Freud's text would suggest. One of the threads that binds him to Dora reappears with increasing visibility as his narrative goes on: it is the problem (or "puzzle," or "riddle," as he calls it) of *where* she learned what she knew. Still more specifically, whether she learned it "orally" or from a book. Moreover, this question is soon linked to another one, that of Dora's relations with women, what Freud calls her "gynaecophilic" currents of feeling (*SE* 7:63, 121 *n.*1; *C* 81, 142 *n.*2). For Freud's defense of his own procedures as dry and "gynaecological" is paralleled by his evocation of the slightly unusual term "gynaecophilic" to describe Dora's homoerotic tendencies: it is as if Freud had a strong interest in clearly marking off the separation of the two realms, in keeping *logos* uncontaminated by *philia*—that is, in defusing the erotic content of acts of knowledge. But for the moment, let us follow the way these two strands—one concerned with the sources of Dora's knowledge of sexual matters, the other with the quality of her gynecophilia—become entangled in Freud's account.

There is, first of all, the governess, "an unmarried woman, no longer young, who is well-read and of advanced views" and of whom Freud remarks in a footnote: "For some time I looked upon this woman as the source of all Dora's secret knowledge, and perhaps I was not entirely wrong in this" (SE 7:36 *n.*1; *C* 52 *n.*21). Perhaps not entirely wrong but not, to his own satisfaction, entirely correct either. For in addition to this person, "with whom Dora had first enjoyed the closest interchange of thought" (SE 7:61; *C* 78) there are others whose effects must be calculated: the "younger of her two cousins," with whom she "had shared all sorts of secrets" (SE 7:61; *C* 78) and, of course, Frau K., with whom she "had lived for years on a footing of the closest intimacy. . . . There was nothing they had not talked about" (SE 7:61; *C* 79). As Freud pursues these matters to more or less of a resolution, it may seem that the question of where Dora learned about sex was merely instrumental—a way of getting at more important material about whom Dora loved. Freud reasons that Dora would not have been so vague—so positively amnesiac—about the sources of her knowledge if she were not trying to protect someone; hence he worries the question of sources so as to press toward a discovery about "object-relations."

The process is summarized in his final footnote, which begins:

> The longer the interval of time that separates me from the end of this analysis, the more probable it seems to me that the fault in my technique lay in this omission: I failed to discover in time and to inform the patient that her homosexual (gynaecophilic) love for Frau K. was the strongest unconscious current in her mental life. I ought to have guessed that the main source of her knowledge of sexual matters could have been no one but Frau K. (*SE* 7:120 *n.*1; *C*, 142 *n.*2)

But this note, with its slightly redundant allusion to "gynaecophilia," rehearses interpretations Freud had set down sixty pages earlier, just before he turned to analyze Dora's two dreams. There, too, he had located Frau K. as both the source of Dora's knowledge and the reason for her forgetfulness, and there, too, he had concluded that "masculine, or, more properly speaking, gynaecophilic currents of feeling are to be regarded as typical of the unconscious erotic life of hysterical girls" (*SE* 7:63; *C* 81). What has transpired in the intervening sixty pages? To begin with, the close analysis of the two dreams—that is, the demonstration of the particular feature of psychoanalytic technique that had prompted the publication of the case history in the first place. But also, in the course of that demonstration, and always in relation to specific associations—sometimes Dora's, sometimes his own—Freud has continued teasing the matter of oral as opposed to written sources, teasing it in ways that seem no longer appropriate once he had formulated his conclusions about Frau K. (*SE* 7:62–63; *C* 80–81), and that, moreover, are presented in a condensed, repetitive, and confusing fashion in these later pages. One is led to suspect that, as Freud would say, "other trains of thought" are operative in fixing his attention on this subject, and it is to them I wish to turn now.

VEHEMENT DISTINCTIONS

Steven Marcus has drawn attention to some passages of bizarre writing in the "Fragment of an Analysis," passages expressing what he calls "fantasies of omniscience, where the demon of interpretation is riding [Freud]" (see essay 3). They occur as Freud is zeroing in on what he takes to be one of Dora's most closely guarded secrets, her childhood masturbation, and in the immediate context of his confronting her with the meaning of a particular "symptomatic act," her fingering the small reticule she wore at her belt. It is worth following Freud's text closely at this point, attending to both the passages Marcus cites and the page of writing that separates them. Marcus' exhibit A is this paragraph of fierce boasting, or gloating:

> There is a great deal of symbolism of this kind in life, but as a rule we pass it by without heeding it. When I set myself the task of bringing to light what human beings keep hidden within them, not by the compelling power of hypnosis, but by observing what they say and what they show, I thought the task was a harder one than it really is. He that has eyes to see and ears to hear may convince himself that no mortal can keep a secret. If his lips are silent, he chatters with his finger-tips; betrayal oozes out of him at every pore. And thus the task of making conscious the most hidden recesses of the mind is one which it is quite possible to accomplish. (*SE* 7:77–78; *C* 96)

Although the vehemence of Freud's tone here is certainly produced by the excitement of his work with Dora, the claims he is making are hyperbolically generalized: "no mortal can keep a secret." In the next paragraph he focuses back on Dora again, and on the details of one particular analytic session: he notices Dora concealing a letter as he enters the room—a letter of no special significance, as it turns out—and concludes that she is signaling, ambivalently, her wish to hold on to her secret. He knows, by now, what that secret is, and because he knows it he can offer to explain to her "her antipathy to every new physician." She is afraid, he tells her, that she will be found out, then immediately contemptuous of the doctors "whose perspicacity she had evidently overestimated before." The situation is defined in adversarial terms: Freud sees himself as one more in a line of "new physicians," but he is determined to be the one who vindicates the profession by successfully extracting Dora's secret. The next sentences celebrate that discovery with a paean of intellectual glee:

> The reproaches against her father for having made her ill, together with the self-reproach underlying them, the leucorrhea, the playing with the reticule, the bed-wetting after her sixth year, the secret which she would not allow the physicians to tear from her—the circumstantial evidence of her having masturbated in childhood—seems to me complete and without a flaw. (*SE* 7:78; *C* 97)

That listing conveys the triumphant sense of wrapping up the package of evidence "complete and without flaw" (in German, *lückenlos*): this is a moment of exuberant intellectual narcissism, of investment in the beautiful totality of one's imaginative product. As such, it is the equivalent of Henry James' fond exclamation about what he had managed to do with Maisie—or with Maisie's help: "I lose myself, truly, in appreciation of my theme." But again, with a difference: for if James' excitement has a Pygmalion quality to it—he has fallen in love with his creation, his theme, and his helpmate—Freud's overflowing fondness can hardly be said to include Dora: if anything, she is diminished by it, seen thoroughly through. Indeed, Freud's ecstasy here might seem totally self-involved with no other object than his own interpretive achievement, if it were not for the sentences that follow, sentences Marcus cites as astonishing instances of "the positive presence of demented and delusional science," a gesture of manic documentation and collegial acknowledgment:

> In the present case I had begun to suspect the masturbation when she had told me of her cousin's gastric pains, and had then identified herself with her by complaining for days together of similar painful sensations. It is well known that gastric pains occur especially often in those who masturbate. According to a personal communication made to me by W. Fliess, it is precisely gastralgias of this character which can be interrupted by an application of co-

caine to the "gastric spot" discovered by him in the nose, and which can be cured by the cauterization of the same spot. (*SE* 7:78; *C* 97)

We might wish to ask whether that "personal communication" was made orally or in writing: Marcus reminds us of the powerful transferential elements at work in Freud's relation to Fliess and suggests that "the case of Dora may also be regarded as part of the process by which Freud began to move toward a resolution of that relation," a relation Freud himself could later characterize as charged with homoerotic feeling. For our purposes what is particularly interesting is the sequence of gestures these paragraphs of Freud's reproduce: the antagonistic, contemptuous pinning down of Dora's secret (significantly, here, it is the secret of self-affection), followed by a giddy celebration of that achievement ("complete and without a flaw"), then *that* inherently unstable moment followed by the hyperbolic ("it is *precisely* gastralgias of this type") and a somewhat beside-the-point invocation of a colleague's expertise, with the homoerotic component that such collegial gestures usually involve here considerably amplified. It is likely that the intensity of Freud's appeal to Fliess is proportionate to the vigor with which he is differentiating himself from Dora, his own mode of knowing from hers; and, by a predictable irony, that intensity leads Freud into a momentary confusion of persons—of himself and his colleague—that resembles the uncertain combination of erotic intimacy and exchanged knowledge Freud detects in Dora's gynecophilic friendships.

For when Freud takes up the question of how much of Dora's knowledge came to her "orally," although he may be primarily tracking down the erotic relations in which she had unconsciously overinvested, following the trail that leads to Frau K., he is also investigating a mode of intercourse that, as we have seen, resembles the oral exchanges of psychoanalytic conversation. We have remarked the care Freud takes to defend the innocence of those exchanges, to insist that, despite their intimate subject matter, they bring him no "gratification." But we may now suspect that there is yet a further danger that he must defend against, the possibility not of sexual misconduct between analyst and patient but of a thoroughgoing epistemological promiscuity in which the lines would blur between what Dora knew and what Freud knew and, consequently, in which the status of Freud's knowledge, and of his professional discourse, would be impugned. In the text of the "Fragment of an Analysis," that danger is figured as the possibility of oral sexual intercourse between two women, the scenario—sensual and discursive at once—that Luce Irigaray was subsequently to call "*quand nos lèvres se parlent,*" "when our lips—the lips of the mouth, the lips of the vagina—speak to each other, speak to themselves, speak among themselves."[4] We can watch Freud at work parrying this threat at one point in his interpretation of Dora's second dream, and doing so by insisting once more on the importance of distinguishing oral and written sources of knowledge. The fragment of the dream being considered is "I then saw a thick wood before me which I went into":

> But she had seen precisely the same thick wood the day before, in a picture at the Secessionist exhibition. In the background of the picture there were *nymphs*.
>
> At this point a certain suspicion of mine became a certainty. The use of "*Bahnhof*" ["station"; literally, "railway-court"] and "*Friedhof*" ["cemetery"; literally, "peace-court"] to represent the female genitals was striking enough in itself, but it also served to direct my awakened curiosity to the similarly formed "*Vorhof*" ["vestibulum"; literally, "fore-court"]—an anatomical term for a particular region of the female genitals. This might have been no more than a misleading joke. But now, with the addition of "nymphs" visible in the background of a "thick wood," no further doubts could be entertained. Here was a symbolic geography of sex! "Nymphae," as is known to physicians though not to laymen (and even by the former the term is not very commonly used), is the name given to the labia minora, which lie in the background of the "thick wood" of the pubic hair. But anyone who employed such technical names as "vestibulum" and "nymphae" must have derived his knowledge from books, and not from popular ones either, but from anatomical text-books or from an encyclopedia—the common refuge of youth when it is devoured by sexual curiosity. If this interpretation were correct, therefore, there lay concealed behind the first situation in the dream a phantasy of defloration, the phantasy of a man seeking to force an entrance into the female genitals. (*SE* 7:99; *C* 119–20)

What is puzzling here is the line of reasoning developed in the last three sentences. Dora's knowing what "nymphae" means may indeed show that she has more than a layman's acquaintance with such "technical" terms, and that, in turn, may betray her reading of encyclopedias; but why should this lead Freud to glimpse a fantasy of defloration or serve as supplementary evidence for the existence of such a fantasy? What does the "therefore" of the last sentence point to? "Anyone who employed such technical names. . . . must have derived *his* knowledge from books": is the shift to the masculine pronoun a way of suggesting that such reading habits, although indulged in by women, are essentially masculine, and hence coordinate with male fantasies of defloration? That would seem to be the logic of this passage; if so, the suggestion that Dora's imagining of the female genitals is bound to be from a man's point of view is of a piece with Freud's persistence in characterizing Dora's love for Frau K. as "masculine." I don't think this is a sign that Freud was squeamish about lesbian love but rather that he was anxious to preserve certain clarities in his thinking about the transfer of psychoanalytic knowledge. It required a vigilant effort, it would seem, to draw the line between the operations in the hysteric, which produce the text of her illness, and those in the analyst, which seek to interpret and dissolve that text, between the production of secrets and the deployment of techniques.

BELATED KNOWLEDGE AND SEX ROLES

Consider the standard account of the relation among hysterical symptoms, secrets, and sexuality: an infantile practice, most often masturbatory, is repressed throughout the latency period, then reappears at puberty, converted into a symptom. What Dora knows, what is written in her physical symptoms, she only knows unconsciously and after the fact, *nachträglich,* and if she is to come to know it consciously, she needs the help of an interlocutor. But what of Freud's knowledge? How did he come by it, and what was the rhythm of its acquisition? Some pages from the beginning of *The History of the Psychoanalytic Movement* offer an intriguing answer. The pages are unusual in a number of respects: unlike the rest of that book, they are not just historical but anecdotal. The narrative powers one sees at work in the "Fragment of an Analysis" are here displayed in miniature, elaborating three brief stories, each with its punch line, that could have appeared in his study of *Witz.* Indeed, they convey the verve—undiminished with repetition—of the inveterate teller of jokes: they sound like stories Freud told again and again and again, bits of autobiographical mythmaking. Their subject: the origins of the "new and original idea" that the neuroses had a sexual etiology, or "How I Stumbled on Psychoanalysis." Their fascination lies in the image of himself Freud chooses to present: here he is neither Conquistador nor Impassive Scientist, but Impressionable Junior Colleague. In that role, he finds himself participating in a drama whose temporal structure is that of the belated surfacing of unconsciously acquired knowledge. Here is how Freud introduces the stories:

> There was some consolation for the bad reception accorded to my contention of a sexual aetiology in the neuroses even by my most intimate circle of friends—for a vacuum rapidly formed itself about my person—in the thought that I was taking up the fight for a new and original idea. But, one day, certain memories gathered in my mind which disturbed this pleasing notion, but which gave me in exchange a valuable insight into the processes of human creative activity and the nature of human knowledge. The idea for which I was being made responsible had by no means originated with me. It had been imparted to me by three people whose opinion had commanded my deepest respect—by Breuer himself, by Charcot, and by Chrobak, the gynaecologist at the University, perhaps the most eminent of all our Vienna physicians. These three men had all communicated to me a piece of knowledge which, strictly speaking, they themselves did not possess. Two of them later denied having done so when I reminded them of the fact: the third (the great Charcot) would probably have done the same if it had been granted me to see him again. But these three identical opinions, which I had heard without understanding, had lain dormant in my mind for years, until one day they awoke in the form of an apparently original discovery. (*SE* 14:12–13)

"These three men had all communicated to me a piece of knowledge which, strictly speaking, they themselves did not possess": questions of possession are important here, of the possibility of possessing knowledge, of "having" an idea, and of the degree of honor, or infamy, that goes with such possessing. Freud, who has experienced what it feels like to be "made responsible" for a disagreeable idea, might wish to share the onus, if not the honor. But he is still more interested in dramatizing the "valuable insight" for which he has—involuntarily, to be sure—exchanged his claim to originality, an insight he finds at once exhilarating, profoundly serviceable, and not a little dismaying: like those jokes he calls "skeptical jokes," it is an insight that might seem to undermine "not a person or an institution but the certainty of our knowledge itself, one of our speculative possessions" (*"Jokes and Their Relation to the Unconscious," SE* 8:115). Here is his account of the first sowing of the seed:

One day, when I was a young house-physician, I was walking across the town with Breuer, when a man came up who evidently wanted to speak to him urgently. I fell behind. As soon as Breuer was free, he told me in his friendly, instructive way that this man was the husband of a patient of his and had brought him some news of her. The wife, he added, was behaving in such a peculiar way in society that she had been brought to him for treatment as a nervous case. He concluded: "These things are always *secrets d'alcôve!"* I asked him in astonishment what he meant, and he answered by explaining the word *alcôve* ("marriage bed") to me, for he failed to realize how extraordinary the *matter* of his statement seemed to me. (*SE* 14:13)

The distribution of roles that will prevail in all three stories is set here: Breuer is the master, friendly and instructive, an older man whose worldliness allows him to sprinkle his speech with bits of French innuendo; Freud is the "young house physician," deferential, grateful for Breuer's attention, still capable of the "astonishment" of the sexually naive, a country boy, *ein Mann vom Lande,* in Kafka's phrase. There is a hint that his astonishment might be, finally, more valuable than the more sophisticated obtuseness that keeps Breuer from realizing how extraordinary what he is saying might seem to his colleague. But this is just a hint: the emphasis is on the *contre-temps.* The value of Freud's "freshness," his Maisie-like capacity to "wonder" until "appearances in themselves vulgar and empty enough . . . begin to have meanings, aspects, solidities, connexions," remains to be brought out more dramatically in the next anecdote:

Some years later, at one of Charcot's evening receptions, I happened to be standing near the great teacher at a moment when he appeared to be telling Brouardel a very interesting story about something that had happened during his day's work. I hardly heard the beginning, but gradually my attention was seized by what he was talking of: a young married couple from a distant country in the East—the woman a severe sufferer, the man either impotent or exceedingly awkward. *"Tâchez donc,"* I heard Charcot repeating, *"je vous assure, vous y arriverez."* Brouardel, who spoke less loudly, must have expressed his astonishment that symptoms like the wife's could have been produced by such circumstances. For Charcot suddenly broke out with great animation: *"Mais, dans des cas pareils c'est toujours la chose génitale, toujours . . . toujours . . . toujours";* and he crossed his arms over his stomach, hugging himself and jumping up and down in his own characteristically lively way. I know that for a moment I was almost paralysed with amazement and said to myself: "Well, but if he knows that, why does he never say so?" But the impression was soon forgotten; brain anatomy and the experimental induction of hysterical paralyses absorbed all my interest. (*SE* 14:13–14)

This skit is more complicated: now it is Brouardel who is in the position of the astonished junior colleague and Freud, younger still, if off to one side, overhearing fragments of a conversation whose effect on him is still more forceful. Two impressions remain vivid over the years: that of the master "hugging himself and jumping up and down" with the delight of knowing what he knows, a moment analogous to Freud's own exhilaration when he was to exclaim "complete and without a flaw" twenty years later; and the sense of being "almost paralysed with amazement" by what he had just heard. If that shock is registered unconsciously it is nevertheless soon forgotten, replaced, among other things, Freud tells us, by considerations of "hysterical paralyses." We should linger on these two allusions to paralysis, so gratuitously juxtaposed. They would seem to be linked: Freud's distinctly marginal relation to this scene of professional knowingness, almost out of earshot, listening to two men talking—in French, of course—about suggestive matters, *secrets d'alcôve,* locates him close to the position of the woman in his analysis of obscene jokes, just as his being paralysed with amazement aligns him with the (mostly female) victims of hysterical paralysis. In his innocence, in his capacity to receive impressions, he is feminized. Or so he keeps insisting:

A year later, I had begun my medical career in Vienna as a lecturer in nervous diseases, and in everything relating to the aetiology of the neuroses I was still as ignorant and innocent as one could expect of a promising student trained at a university. One day I had a friendly message from Chrobak, asking me to take a woman patient of his to whom he could not give enough time, owing to his new appointment as a university teacher. I arrived at the patient's house before he did and found that she was suffering from attacks of meaningless anxiety, and could only be soothed by the most precise information about where her doctor was at every moment of the day. When Chrobak arrived he took me aside and told me that the patient's anxiety was due to the fact that although she had been married for eighteen years she was still *virgo intacta.* The husband was absolutely impotent. In such cases, he said, there was nothing for a medical man to do but to shield this domestic misfortune with his own reputation, and put up with it if people shrugged their shoulders and said of him: "He's no good if he can't cure her after so many years." The sole prescriptions for such a malady, he added, is familiar enough to us, but we cannot order it. It runs:

R_x Penis normalis
dosim
repetatur!"

I had never heard of such a prescription, and felt inclined to shake my head over my kind friend's cynicism. (*SE* 14:14-15)

"I had never heard of such a prescription": the note of the ingénue is caught in that phrase, but Freud's rueful shake of the head is not quite a gesture of astonishment or amazed paralysis. It is his more settled acknowledgment of a cast of mind he finds cynical, one that has gynecologists aligning themselves with impotent husbands, willing to risk their reputations "to shield this domestic misfortune," although unwilling—or simply unable—to include the wife's "misfortune" as part of the calculation. Freud is not taking a strong polemical stance against these commonplace sexual and medical arrangements, but he is glancing at the structures of complicity, between doctors and husbands, that keep the sexual etiology of the neuroses a well-kept, smoking room secret. His own position is no longer that of the impressionable hysteric, taking in knowledge she will not know she has, but it is still outside the circle of collegiality. Freud presents himself as susceptible to the lures of that primarily male world, flattered for instance, by Chrobak's friendship and patronage, but with more serious intellectual ambitions; his imagery shifts to more masculine resonances:

I have not of course disclosed the illustrious parentage of this scandalous idea in order to saddle other people with the responsibility for it. I am well aware that it is one thing to give utterance to an idea once or twice in the form of a passing *aperçu*, and quite another to mean it seriously—to take it literally and pursue it in the face of every contradictory detail, and to win it a place among accepted truths. It is the difference between a casual flirtation and a legal marriage with all its duties and difficulties. "*Epouser les idées de* . . ." is no uncommon figure of speech, at any rate in French. (SE 14:15)

At this point, Freud is back in the world of men, of Oedipal rivalry, to be precise. Breuer, Charcot, and Chroback have their flirtations with the sexual etiology of the neuroses, but Freud has made an honest woman of her, by his persistence, his intellectual mastery, the stolid virility of his pursuit. But the "idea" that he has wed was—and that is the point of these stories—acquired in a structure of *nachträglichkeit*, analogous to the hysteric's acquisition of her often paralyzing secrets. Freud needs both to acknowledge the strangeness of this procedure—it is his claim, after all, to be taken more seriously than Breuer, Charcot, or Chrobak—and to domesticate the structure, to bring it into the light of conscious reflection, to deploy it as technique.

We have been locating the same ambivalence in Freud's dealings with Dora. For the session-by-session acquisition of knowledge about his patients, in the interplay of their (oral) free associations and his own free-floating attention and (oral) interventions, is governed by the same rhythms of unconscious, latent acquisition, of overhearing, that Freud has dramatized in these stories about his original discovery. Just as in those anecdotes he seems to be running the risk of feminization, so in the "Fragment of an Analysis" he would seem, at points, to be fending off whatever reminds him of the possibility that such oral intercourse is regressive, epistemologically unstable. He is not speaking lightly when he says, toward the end of his case history, that it would have been "quite impracticable . . . to deal simultaneously with the technique of analysis and with the internal structure of a case of hysteria" (*SE* 7:112; *C* 134). The matter of Dora and the matter of the techniques that are brought into touch with her symptoms and words are quite literally out of phase in Freud's thinking; they have to be, he believes, if he is to claim scientific status for those techniques and the discoveries that prompted them. The mistakes Freud made in his sessions with Dora and the misconstructions he permitted himself in writing the case up suggest that, among other things, Dora was sacrificed to underwrite that claim.

Notes

1. Henry James, Preface to "What Maisie Knew," in *The Art of the Novel*, R. P. Blackmur, ed (New York: Scribner, 1934), pp. 148–49.

2. Philip Rieff, *Fellow Teachers* (New York: Harper & Row, 1973), p. 84. Rieff was the first to point out, as far as I know, the resemblance of Maisie and Dora: "Alas, poor Dora: there were no longer truths strong enough in her resistances to fight off, unsupported, the assaults of experience. Dora had no protector against the deadly competitive erotic circles that drew themselves around her. Unlike Maisie's author, the spiritual author of Dora could think of everything except to support those resistant, self-perpetuating truths by which Dora's neurotic, self-divided, and socially isolated resistances were once chartered. Freud's special mission was to point out to Dora the fact (which is changeable, like all facts—changeable, not least, by the authority of his interpretation) that her truths had become neurotic, mere resistances signaling their opponents, her desires" (p. 85). These sentences convey some sense both of Rieff's central concern—the erosion of moral authority, an erosion accelerated by Freud's "interpretations"—and of the densely ironic style in which this strange book is elaborated.

3. It is worth noticing the vicissitudes of this word in Freud's writings. Most often it is used in phrases like "the technique of dream interpretation" or "the technique of psychoanalysis" to suggest certain procedures available to the analyst. But in Freud's book on *Witz*, published in 1905, the year he was revising the "Fragment of an Analysis" for publication, he uses "technique" and its cognates steadily to mean the mechanisms that produce the joke, not the means of its interpretation; so the word crosses the line and becomes synonomous with "joke work" (a term Freud employs much less frequently) and homologous with "dream work" and the work of producing symptoms, that is, with "the internal structure of the neurosis." At this point, "techniques" and "secrets" begin to look alike.

4. Luce Irigaray, *Ce sexe qui n'en est pas un* (Paris: Minuit, 1977), pp. 205–17.

11. Questioning the Unconscious: The Dora Archive

JERRE COLLINS, J. RAY GREEN, MARY LYDON, MARK SACHNER, ELEANOR HONIG SKOLLER

Others abide our question. Thou art free.
Matthew Arnold

What is involved in the recording and narration of history? This question is one of the most important posed by the Dora archive. Freud acknowledges as much when he writes, in the opening pages of this, his first psychoanalytic case history: "The presentation of my case histories remains a problem which is hard for me to solve," and again: "Indeed I have not yet succeeded in solving the problem of how to record for publication the history of a treatment of long duration" (*SE* 7:10; *C* 24). This problem manifests itself in the Dora case history in a number of ways. To begin with, Freud displays reticence both by withholding information about the case and by withholding the case history itself from publication for five years. In addition, Freud could not record immediately or remember later everything that occurred in the analysis, a fact he acknowledges. He acknowledges too that in order to fill in the gaps of his memory he has recourse to material from other cases. Furthermore, he misremembers at least once, insisting in a note added in 1923 that the treatment was broken off on the last day of

This essay was first published in *Diacritics* (Spring 1983), pp. 37–42.

1899, whereas it actually ended one year later, as a letter to Fliess (dated January 25, 1901) indicates. Finally, in his redaction of the case history, he does not present the material in the order in which it was given in the course of the analysis. This reordering is initially presented as a deliberate strategy: "Nothing of any importance has been altered in it except in some places the order in which the explanations are given; and this has been done for the sake of presenting the case in a more connected form" (*SE,* 7:10; *C,* 24). The reordering, however, is sometimes involuntary. When it is voluntary, Freud justifies it on the grounds of his concern for the demands of narrative. When it is involuntary, he apologizes, as at the end of the case history, for "the somewhat haphazard order" in which he presents the analysis of Dora's second dream (*SE* 7:95; *C* 115). And it is precisely the most recent material, the material that should be freshest in his memory (but that is most closely connected with the abrupt termination of the case) whose order he is unable to reproduce.

The parallel, unnoticed by Freud, between the above four characteristics of his presentation and what he perceived to be characteristics of the neurotic's discourse in analysis—reticence, amnesia, paramnesia, and alteration of chronology—is striking. He writes:

The patients' inability to give an ordered history of their life in so far as it coincides with the history of their illness is not merely characteristic of the neurosis. It also possesses great theoretical significance. For this inability has the following grounds. In the first place, patients consciously and intentionally keep back part of what they ought to tell—things that are perfectly well known to them—because they have not got over their feelings of timidity and shame (or discretion, where what they say concerns other people); this is the share taken by *conscious* disingenuousness. In the second place, part of the anamnestic knowledge, which the patients have at their disposal at other times, disappears while they are actually telling their story, but without their making any deliberate reservations: the share taken by *unconscious* disingenuousness. In the third place, there are invariably true amnesias—gaps in the memory into which not only old recollections but even quite recent ones have fallen—and paramnesias, formed secondarily so as to fill in those gaps. When the events themselves have been kept in mind, the purpose underlying the amnesias can be fulfilled just as surely by destroying a connection, and a connection is most surely broken by altering the chronological order of events. The latter always proves to be the most vulnerable element in the store of memory and the one which is most easily subject to repression. Again, we meet with many recollections that are in what might be described as the first stage of repression, and these we find surrounded with doubts. At a later period the doubts would be replaced by a loss or a falsification of memory. (SE 7:16–17; *C* 31–32)

Although Freud recognizes the "great theoretical significance" of these tactics in the discourse of the neurotic, he overlooks their theoretical significance and even their very presence in his own discourse. Rather than conclude from the presence of these tactics that Freud himself is neurotic, as some have done, we find it more useful to focus on the theoretical significance of his blindness, to view it as evidence of the problematic nature of the very notion of a privileged position, a position from which judgments can be made while remaining itself exempt from judgment. Hence, for example, Lacan's insistence on the implication of the analyst in the analysis—but even Lacan privileges a certain Freud. The question must be raised, therefore, of whether it is possible to develop a language of interpretation that does not demand the adoption of a privileged position at least provisionally. The dynamic of interpretation bedevils all who venture to interpret, not only Freudians. Yet we must not forget that it is Freud's analytic technique that enables us to see that interpretation is a "knife that cuts both ways," that is to say, even though interpretation is always overdetermined, even though it includes unconscious and conscious determinants, one must nonetheless interpret.

Within Freud's analytic technique, however, there is one tactic that has aroused the indignation of many of his critics, feminist critics in particular. Freud describes this stratagem and the situation which gives rise to it as follows:

When a patient brings forward a sound and incontestable train of argument during psychoanalytic treatment, the physician is liable to feel a moment's embarrassment, and the patient may take advantage of it by asking: "This is all perfectly correct and true, isn't it? What do you want to change in [it] now that I've told you?" But it soon becomes evident that the patient is using thoughts of this kind, which the analysis cannot attack, for the purpose of cloaking others which are anxious to escape from criticism and from consciousness. A string of reproaches against other people leads one to suspect the existence of a string of self-reproaches with the same content. All that need be done is to turn back each particular reproach on to the speaker himself. (*SE* 7:35; *C* 51)

The juxtaposition of the notion of "a sound and incontestable train of argument" with "a string of reproaches against other people" in the quotation above bears a striking similarity to the structure of Freud's Prefatory Remarks to Dora's case history, in which he is equally preoccupied with constructing a coherent narrative and with expressing misgivings about his readers. He denounces his readers before the fact for the reproaches he anticipates from them on two counts: the betrayal of a patient's confidence and perhaps of her identity as well, and the frank discussion of sexual matters with a young girl.[1]

Freud's analytic technique with Dora involved refusing to accept at face value Dora's "sound and incontestable train of argument," reversing the reproaches against her father to reveal a hidden self-reproach on her part, and using the self-reproach to point to a further explanation, which the logical argument was designed to protect. Rather than attacking Dora's insight into her position as "object for barter" (*SE* 7:34; *C* 50), Freud reverses her reproaches against her father to reveal the self-reproach that she had from the beginning been complicit in the affair between her father and Frau K. He then uses this self-reproach to suggest another logical and coherent explanation that is less complimentary and more troublesome to Dora. What particularly angers the critics here is that precisely the most logical and coherent statements of the patient are undermined. In Dora's case these statements relate to her position as pawn in the nexus of relationships between the K. family and her own. What is particuarly irksome to Freud's critics is that, although he admits the accuracy of Dora's explanation, he nonetheless discounts it. It is Freud's belief in the existence of the unconscious that divides him from his critics. What these critics do not see is that if the unconscious exists, then Freud's own narrative is subject to unconscious determinants. Furthermore, Freud's narrative, employing as it does the same tactics as Dora's, is therefore susceptible to analysis by the same stratagem.

Behind the reproaches Freud directs to his readers lies a hidden self-reproach precisely for betraying Dora's secrets and for speaking frankly to her about sexual matters. As for Freud's own "sound and incontestable train of argument" that the case foundered because he did not "succeed in mastering the transference in good time (*SE* 7:118; *C* 140), meaning here Dora's identification of him with Herr K., we would argue, following Freud's technique, that while this is true, it also functions as a screen interpretation for another explanation less complimentary and more troublesome to Freud himself. Besides the "unknown quantity in me which reminded Dora of Herr K." (*SE* 7:119; *C* 141) which Freud could accept, there was also a quantity unknown to him that reminded Dora of Frau K. Who is it in Dora's story, after all, who both speaks frankly to her about sex and betrays her confidence? If it was true that Dora's homosexual love for Frau K. was "the strongest unconscious current in her mental life" (*SE* 7:120, *n.*1; *C* 142, *n.*2), it is equally true, we suggest, that Dora's identification of Freud with Frau K. in the transference was an aspect of the analysis so difficult for Freud to accept that he failed even to acknowledge it.

What is significant here is Freud's refusal of identification with Frau K. as the object of "Dora's deep-rooted homosexual love" (*SE* 7:105, *n.*2; *C* 125, *n.*20), and not simply his reluctance to acknowledge that Frau K. is that object. Let us examine the structure of Freud's text. Twice, once in each of the last two sections of the book, Freud juxtaposes a discussion involving Herr K. with a footnote having to do, wholly or in part, with Frau K. In both cases the Sistine Madonnna, which Dora saw in Dresden, functions as a bridge between the two. In the first instance there is in a footnote a lengthy analysis of the importance of the Madonna for Dora, an analysis that seems unconnected either to what precedes or to what follows. At the end of the section on the second dream, after analyzing Dora's fantasy of childbirth, Freud convinces her of the persistence of her love for Herr K. ("And Dora disputed the fact no longer" [*SE* 7:104; *C* 125]). Following this observation there is a long footnote in which Freud amends his interpretation, suggesting that behind Herr K. there lies another and more troublesome love object. He declares in the analysis of the second dream that "behind the almost limitless series of displacements . . .

brought to light, it was possible to divine the operation of a single simple factor—Dora's deep-rooted homosexual love for Frau K." (*SE* 7:104, *n.* 2; *C* 125, *n.* 20).

In the second instance, the reference to the Madonna is in the text and is clearly linked on the one hand to the transference and on the other hand to Dora's rejection of men and her homosexual attachment to Frau K. Just as in the first juxtaposition the text deals with Herr K. as Dora's love-object, in the second it deals with him as the source of the transference. One might expect the second footnote, then, to deal with Frau K. as source of the transference and the following schema to hold:

text:	Herr K.	love object	transference
footnotes:	Frau K.	love object	transference

In fact, however, the second footnote does not link Frau K. with the transference (and Freud's failure to "master" it) at all but only reiterates the earlier observation that Frau K. was Dora's love-object. In the second juxtaposition, Freud gives two reasons for the abrupt termination of the analysis, one in the text, one in the footnote. He seems to be setting up a parallel, even on the level of language ("I did not succeed . . . in good time" [*SE* 7:118; *C* 140] in the text, "I failed to discover in time" [*SE* 7:120, *n.* 1; *C* 142, *n.* 2] in the footnote). But the reason given in the footnote is not credible since it ignores everything he had learned about analysis and the transference even by 1905. He writes:

> The longer the interval of time that separates me from the end of this analysis, the more probable it seems to me that the fault in my technique lay in this omission: I failed to discover in time and to inform the patient that her homosexual (gynaecophilic) love for Frau K. was the strongest current in her mental life.

Yet Freud had long since abandoned the notion that it was sufficient for the analyst to inform the patient of the contents of her unconscious to effect a cure. He came to realize that the patient's strong resistances to making conscious what had been unconscious must be overcome and that, as he put it in 1912, analysis was "a situation in which finally every conflict has to be fought out in the sphere of transference" ("The Dynamics of Transference," *SE* 12:104). In effect the second footnote is an astonishing repression of the notion of transference. What is the motivation for this repression? Is it not Freud's inability to accept identification not merely with a woman but with a woman who is the object of a love that is homosexual? We suggest that this question might lead straight to the explanation that is less complimentary and more troublesome to Freud, the rock on which the analysis of Dora really foundered.

It is necessary at this point to return to the figure of the Madonna, which so fascinated Dora and which Freud chose to insert as a middle term between Herr K. and Frau K. Freud asserts:

> The *"Madonna"* was obviously Dora herself; in the first place because of the "adorer" who had sent her the pictures, in the second place because she had won Herr K.'s love chiefly by the motherliness she had shown towards his children, and lastly because she had had a child though she was still a girl (this being a direct allusion to the phantasy of childbirth). (*SE* 7:104, *n.* 2: *C* 125, *n.* 20)

Dora's identification with the Virgin Mother thus reflects at once her yearning for motherhood and her repudiation of men. "Men are all so detestable that I would rather not marry. This is my revenge" (*SE* 7:120; *C* 142) is Freud's rendering of a central dream thought in Dora's second dream. But can the significance of the Madonna be so simply exhausted? Is there not beneath Freud's explanation yet another?

In the second dream Dora attempts unsuccessfully to return to her mother; indeed she goes home, only to find her mother absent. This places Dora's contemplation of the Sistine Madonna in another perspective. Her immobilization in front of this image recalls the fascination of the mirror-stage, in which the child is held in its mother's arms before its own reflection.[2] It may be, therefore, that Dora's deepest desire is not identification with the mother (in the sense of the assumption of the mother's role) but fusion with the mother, a return to that "desperate paradise" which is riven by entry into the Symbolic.[3] Indeed, late in his career Freud even suggested that there was an intimate relationship between an unresolved attachment to the mother and the etiology of hysteria (*SE* 21:227).

Freud chooses to see Dora's leaving him as an acting out of her desire for revenge on Herr K., who had dismissed her; in other words, he recognizes finally the transference from Herr K. We submit that beneath this explanation lies another, that her leaving is a repetition of her "dismissal" of her mother and that behind her transference from Frau K., which Freud never really recognizes, there is an even more occulted transference from her mother. The Madonna, which Freud uses as a middle term between Herr K. and Frau K., Dora uses as a middle term between her mother and Freud. Even Freud notices that he is being linked to the Madonna: "At the time she was telling me the dream I was still unaware . . . that we had only *two hours* more work before us. This was the same length of time which she had spent in front of the Sistine Madonna" (*SE* 7:119; *C* 141). But he draws no further conclusions from this. Freud's refusal to pursue his link with the Madonna is telling. Had he pursued it, he might have been able to see Dora's neurotic conflict and its emergence in the transference in a new light. He might have seen that what she most desired, and what she neurotically fled, was not the heterosexual relationship (Freud taking the place of Herr K. and ultimately of the father) but the homosexual one (Freud taking the place of Frau K. and ultimately of the mother).[4]

There is one aspect of Dora's version of things that Freud exempts from his questioning, namely her assessment of her mother: "The daughter looked down on the mother and used to criticize her mercilessly, and she had withdrawn completely from her influence" (*SE* 7:20; *C* 34). Freud uncharacteristically accepts this reading at face value and concurs. He writes, "I never made her mother's acquaintance. From the accounts given me by the girl and her father I was led to imagine her as an uncultivated woman and above all as a foolish one" (*SE* 7:20; *C* 34). As Suzanne Gearhart has pointed out, Freud joins Dora in dismissing her mother on these grounds (see essay 5). Throughout the analysis Freud acts as if the mother were of no consequence in Dora's psychic life. Is there not a structural parallel between Freud's complacency on this point and the eclipsing of the mother in the theory of the Oedipus complex? Is it not possible to see the Oedipus complex, which Freud certainly always took to be "a sound and incontestable train of argument," as a screen explanation behind which lies another one less complimentary and more troublesome to him? Freud found aggressive wishes directed toward the father intolerable; in fact, he viewed parricide as the necessary evil upon which civilization is founded. But did he not find intolerable the very notion of aggressive wishes directed toward the mother? If he did, this would elucidate Freud's complicity with Dora in her repression of her mother. But as we have tried to show, this repression on Dora's part conceals a deep involvement with the mother. Might not Freud's parallel occulting of the mother in the Oedipus complex conceal a similar involvement on his part? This hidden preoccupation with the mother could be viewed as an individual phenomenon. But is it not more useful to see this blindness in so astute an analyst as the manifestation in him of a perversion—the repression of the mother—which lies at the root of Western civilization itself?

It is not our intention to reduce the multiple transferences that Lacan and Suzanne Gearhart have recognized and discussed to a "single simple factor," the transference from the father and from the mother. To the extent that there is a "single simple factor," it is a structural one, and the actual historical mother and father are only the first in an "almost limitless series of displacements" (*SE* 7:104, *n.*2; *C* 125, *n.*20). The series expands as new relationships accumulate, and in each new relationship the entire series of transferences from prior relationships comes into play. But some of these transferences are resisted to various degrees, and the constellation of resistances, at least some of them unconscious, is called countertransference. As Lacan puts it: "What is this transference after all . . . ? Cannot it be considered to be an entity entirely relative to the countertransference defined as the sum of the prejudices, the passions, the difficulties . . . of the analyst at a given moment of the dialectical process?"[5] But perhaps it is not so much the transference as the recognition of the transference that is relative to the countertransference. Freud could not recognize the transference from Frau K., so instead of reproducing it in the analysis, he acts it out, thereby doing precisely what he accuses Dora of having done: "Thus she *acted out* an essential part of her recollections and phantasies instead of reproducing it in the treatment" (*SE* 7:119; *C* 141). Like Frau K., Freud speaks frankly with Dora about sexual matters and he betrays her confidence.[6]

Outside the limitations of the analytic situation, which are intended to restrict the analysand to transferences and the analyst to counter-transference, each individual enters a relationship with her or his repertoire of transferences and her or his constellation of resistances.

But Freud is not simply a replica of Herr K. or of any of the others from whom Dora forms her transferences. Besides the "unknown quantity" in him that reminded Dora of Herr K., besides the unknown quantity that reminded her of Frau K., there is a further unknown quantity in Freud that has nothing to do with any of Dora's transferences and is in excess of them. The total of these unknown quantities constitutes the historical subject: Sigmund Freud. It is only scrupulous attention to the concrete historicity of the other that can reveal something beyond the expectations provoked by the transferences. In the case of Freud, for example, the only way out of the hall of mirrors of multiple transferences is by constant appeal to that Freud who is in excess of them. Indeed, in any relationship the only escape from the hall of mirror is through a constant attempt to make contact with that in the other which is in excess of the transferences, even though the unknown quantity in the other, to the extent that it is in excess of the transferences, cannot be recognized, cannot be known.[7] Knowledge beyond the transferences is a knowledge of difference, a knowledge that there is something in the other that one cannot recognize, that escapes one's grasp.

Notes

1. But Freud was not always as frank as he claimed. In spite of his assertion that "the best way of speaking of such things is to be dry and direct," he refers to oral sex as "sexual gratification *per os*," resorting to Latin, perhaps to avoid the connection with the "oral source" of Dora's information about sex, Frau K., while he resorts to

French maxims to describe the very technique of being dry and direct: "J'appelle un chat un chat" and "pour faire une omelette il faut casser des oeufs" (*SE* 7:48–49; *C* 65–66).

2. One might also note that the first juxtaposition in which the Madonna is inserted as a bridge between Herr K. and Frau K. involves a discussion of Dora's love object(s). Freud's insertion of the Madonna into this context seems incongruous, since he mentions only Dora's identification with her. But the complete juxtaposition (Herr K., Madonna, Frau K.) suggests that the Freudian unconscious knew more than the Freudian conscious would admit.

3. Jeffrey Mehlman, *A Structural Study of Autobiography* (Ithaca: Cornell University Press, 1974), p. 25.

4. Perhaps this would illuminate the characteristic behavior of neurotics as Freud describes it: "Incapacity for meeting a real erotic demand is one of the essential features of a neurosis. Neurotics are dominated by the opposition between reality and phantasy. If what they long for the most intensely in their phantasies is presented to them in reality, they none the less flee from it" (*SE* 7:110; *C* 132). Insofar as the neurotic sees erotic satisfaction not as a substitute for but as a replication of the original state of fusion, her/his flight is logical, for fusion entails dissolution of the self.

5. Jacques Lacan, *Ecrits,* Alan Sheridan tr. (New York: Norton, 1977), p. 116. (For Rose translation, see essay 4).

6. Why does Freud not recognize until the analysis is safely over that Frau K. was the "oral source" of Dora's sexual knowledge? He had the information necessary for the inference from the very beginning of the case. In her father's summary of Dora's history, given to Freud before he began treating her, Freud learned that Herr K., in his defensive response to Dora's report of his proposition, "proceeded to throw suspicion upon the girl, saying that he had heard from Frau K. that she took no interest in anything but sexual matters, and that she used to read Mantegazza's *Physiology of Love* and books of that sort in their house on the lake" (*SE* 7:26; *C* 41). Frau K. knew too much not to be implicated in Dora's knowledge. Perhaps Freud's inability to draw an obvious conclusion here was part of his resistance to the transference from Frau K.

With regard to Freud's resistance to transference from the mother, see his remark to H. D.: " 'I must tell you . . . I do not *like* to be the mother in transference—it always surprises and shocks me a little. I feel very masculine.' I asked him if others had what he called this mother-transference on him. He said ironically and I thought a little wistfully, 'O, very many.' " H. D., *Tribute to Freud* (1956; New York: McGraw-Hill, 1975), p. 146.

7. Is this not the grain of truth in Freud's curious statement that would appear, as J. Rose says, to undermine "the whole discovery of psychoanalysis" (see essay 6) that "it is possible for a neurosis to be overcome by reality" (*SE* 7:110; *C* 132)?

12. Enforcing Oedipus: Freud and Dora

MADELON SPRENGNETHER

Philip Rieff, in his introduction to Freud's "Fragment of an Analysis of a Case of Hysteria," refers to the intricately structured love life of Dora's family as a "group illness" (*C* 10). More specifically, he points out that "the sick daughter has a sick father, who has a sick mistress, who has a sick husband, who proposes himself to the sick daughter as her lover. Dora does not want to hold hands in this charmless circle—although Freud does, at one point, indicate that she should." At another point in his discussion of Freud's narrative technique he comes close to admitting that Freud himself participates in the "neurotic eroticism" of this domestic scene. Having noted Freud's nonlinear, novelistic technique, he speculates briefly that "Freud's own therapeutic habits—spinning out beautiful and complicated lines of argument—meet all the requirements of neurotic brilliance," choosing however not to pursue this line of reasoning (*C* 19). More recent readers of *Dora* point to the elements of countertransference in this case history, revealing the extent of Freud's subjective involvement in his construction of Dora's responses.[1] In my own reading of *Dora*, I want to consider

This essay appears for the first time. It will be reprinted in *The M/Other Tongue: Essays in Feminist Psychoanalytic Criticism*, Madelon Sprengnether, Shirley Garner, and Claire Kahane, eds. (Ithaca: Cornell University Press, forthcoming).

first the relationship between illness and seduction, then the degree of Freud's complicity in this structure, and finally the ways in which Freud's narrative style may be viewed as symptomatic or hysterical.

PLAYING DOCTOR

The Politics of Naming. Freud himself, in his passion for significance, reveals the genesis of the pseudonym Dora.

Who else was there called Dora? I should have liked to dismiss with incredulity the next thought to occur to me—that it was the name of my sister's nursemaid. . . . I had seen a letter on my sister's dining room table addressed to "Fräulein Rosa W." I asked in surprise who there was of that name, and was told that the girl I knew as Dora was really called Rosa, but had had to give up her real name when she took up employment in the house, since my sister could take the name "Rosa" as applying to herself as well. "Poor people," I remarked in pity, "they cannot even keep their own names!" . . . When next day I was looking for a name for someone *who could not keep her own,* "Dora" was the only one to occur to me. (*The Psychopathology of Everyday Life.* (*SE* 12:241)

To this piece of intimate information Steven Marcus adds the association with David Copperfield's invalid child-wife Dora.[2] Both lines of association seem relevant, given the fact that nearly everyone in Dora's family circle occupies the role of nurse or invalid, and sometimes both.

Notable among the ill are: Dora's father, suffering from tuberculosis, syphilis, detached retina, partial paralysis, confusional mental states, and a nervous cough; Frau K., the victim of some form of paralysis, preventing her from being able to walk; Dora's mother, afflicted with a vaginal discharge, presumably gonorrhea contracted from her husband; Dora's aunt, dying from a wasting disease; her uncle, a "hypochondriacal bachelor"; and Dora herself, prey to shortness of breath, coughing, loss of voice, an apparent attack of appendicitis, a catarrh, and a vaginal discharge of undetermined origin. In this atmosphere of real and pretended illness, Dora's mother, about whom we know very little, accepts expensive presents of jewelry from her husband, ignores the relationship between her husband and Frau K., as well as the attentions paid by Herr K. to her daughter, locks doors, and otherwise spends her time in obsessive housecleaning.[3] Significantly, she refuses the role of nurse, which falls first to Dora, whose attachment to her father is based in part on her attentions to him during his various ailments. The extent to which the role of nurse involves service or, more specifically, caretaking links it with that of nursemaid or governess, both positions of subordination and even exploitation in this story. While Dora's governess betrays the affection of her charge in her pursuit of the elusive love of Dora's father, the K.'s governess suffers a worse fate, given the fact that Herr K. first seduces then abandons her. The position of nurse/nursemaid/governess offers only the illusion of control, and it is no accident that Freud associates the position of Ida Bauer in her family with that of his sister's nursemaid, a role that confers seeming maternal power firmly fixed within the context of patriarchal control.[4]

Frau K., moreover, repeats the pattern of Dora's nursing her father, displacing her in the process. From occupying the privileged position of nurse in relation to her father, Dora is abruptly shifted to that of nursemaid or governess, disappointed in her love for the master. Frau K., in the meantime, trades the role of invalid for that of nurse, revealing the extent to which both giving and receiving attention are predicated on illness. Dora's option for the role of invalid might be seen in this light as both a desperate bid for affection and a means of avoiding, temporarily at least, the nurse/governess role, associated in both households with betrayal. Complicating Dora's situation is her role as nursemaid of the K.'s children and her intimacy with Frau K. based on the exclusion of Herr K., until the time of her father's affair. Deprived of the role (involving for her maternal rather than sexual ministrations) on which she had counted for eliciting the affection and attentions of members of both families, Dora, now excluded by her father and Frau K., is offered only one position, that of Herr K.'s mistress, rendering her powerless and vulnerable to further rejection. Freud's choice of a name for Dora would seem to fix her in her dilemma.

Freud performs another significant act of naming in regard to Dora, attributing to her the specific sexual fantasy of fellatio. The choice of this fantasy is central, I believe, not only to Freud's subsequent interpretations of Dora's unconscious wishes, but also to the stance he adopts toward her in his narrative.

If there is a "primal scene" in this narrative it is not the classic one in which the child imagines a sadistic father inflicting pain on his mother. The scene of seduction rather focuses on Dora's father and Frau K. engaged in an act of intercourse, which Freud himself imagines, names, and then at length defends. On the basis of a backward pun (assuming that the phrase *ein vermögender Mann* for Dora means *ein unvermögender Mann*) Freud concludes that Dora's father is impotent.[5] "Dora confirmed this interpretation," he claims, "from her conscious knowledge" (*SE* 7:47; *C* 64), although he does not inquire into the source of such knowledge on her part. Moving quickly, Freud presses Dora to admit that she knows of "more than one way of obtaining sexual gratification." It is Freud's conclusion that fellatio is the primary means of sexual gratification employed by Dora's father and Frau K. and that it is precisely this fantasy that preoccupies Dora, giving rise to one of her hysterical symptoms, the state of irritation of her throat and her oral cavity. What is curious here is that Freud imagines a scene in which a woman gives sexual solace to a man, but not the reverse. If it is true that Dora's reading of Mantegazza's *Physiology of Love* has given her knowledge of the practice of fellatio, then it would make sense to suppose that she had equal knowledge of cunnilingus.[6] If it is also true that Frau K. and Dora have shared intimacies about Frau K.'s sexual life with her husband, from whom Frau K. witholds herself, preferring to share her bedroom with Dora, and that they have read Mantegazza together, then it would make even more sense that Dora's fantasy life (if it includes fellatio) would also include cunnilingus. Full sexual gratification, moreover, supposing the impotence of Dora's father, is more easily imaginable for the woman with this fantasy than it is with the one Freud proposes. At this important juncture in his interpretation of Dora's hysterical symptoms, Freud chooses, despite her unwillingness to confirm his theory, to maintain that Dora fantasizes fellatio. This fantasy then becomes the cornerstone of his subsequent interpretations of Dora's repressed love for Herr K. Let us look, then, at some of the determinants of this crucial choice.

The fantasied scene of seduction in Dora's family, according to Freud, is one in which Dora gives sexual satisfaction, in the form of fellatio, to her impotent father (*SE* 7:48, 83; *C* 65, 102). This fantasy is remarkable not only in terms of its incestuous character but also in the way in which it reproduces the structure of the nurse-invalid relationship. Dora's father, by occupying the role of invalid, a curiously passive stance in relation to Freud's orthodox notions of male heterosexuality, compels his partner into the role of nurse, so that the act of fellatio appears as one more ministration to his need. At the same time, the figure of the nursemaid, ever present in this case history, recurs oddly in Freud's defense of his discussion of this "perversion" (*SE* : 7:51; *C* 67). In a brilliant series of analogies, Freud relates fellatio regressively to thumbsucking and ultimately to breastfeeding, culminating in the following observation.

> It then needs very little creative power to substitute the sexual object of the moment (the penis) for the original object (the nipple) or for the finger which does duty for it, and to place the current sexual object in the situation in which gratification was originally obtained. So we see that this excessively repulsive and perverted phantasy of sucking at a penis has the most innocent origin. It is a new version of what may be described as a prehistoric impression of sucking at the mother's or a nurse's breast—an impression which has usually been revived by contact with children who are being nursed. In most instances a cow's udder has aptly played the part of an image intermediate between a nipple and a penis. (*SE* 7:52; *C* 69–70)

By the end of this passage there is no clear line of demarcation between the nurser and the nurse. Frau K. in her sexual activity with Dora's father may be said to "nurse" him in two different senses, both of which "feminize" her partner, either through identification with the figure of the passive invalid or through that of the nursemaid who breastfeeds her charge. The image of the cow's udder, a shape that mediates between the nipple and the penis, marks the ground of this indeterminacy.

Freud's choice of a name and of a fantasy for Dora lock her into an apparently subordinate relationship to the object of love. The conjunction of love and illness in the scene of seduction, however, creates a paradoxical source of power in the figure of the nurse. The primary figure in this fantasy is female, just as the primary organ may be said to be the nipple rather than the penis. Against this image of fluid gender identity, Freud constructs a more conventional scene of heterosexual seduction, one that he then presses Dora to accept. Freud's "interpretation" of Dora's repressed love of Herr K. serves at least two functions. It permits the nurse–invalid structure of sexual relations to survive as a fantasy along with the surrender of an aggressive male role, at the same time that it denies the power of the figure of the nurse, by asserting the more culturally sanctioned role division in the structure of Herr K.'s relation to Dora. If the first structure may be described as preoedipal, focusing as it does on a maternal figure, the second is clearly oedipal. The oedipal overlay is the one with which Freud himself identifies, effectively preventing him from exploring the extent to which he also identifies with the figure of the nurse, or with the feminine position generally, which he tends to associate with homosexuality.[7] The power of the nurse to disrupt Freud's oedipal interpretation persists, however, through refusal, which Freud understands as rejection and ultimately as "revenge." The conflict between the two levels of fantasy in this case history repeats itself in the form of the narrative, appearing symptomatically as Freud's anxiety about filling gaps and completeness.

While Freud displays, from time to time, a skeptical attitude toward Dora's father, admitting to the validity of some of Dora's claims about his lack of straightforwardness, he is remarkably uncritical of Herr K., whom he considers to be an attractive lover.[8] In the two instances in which Herr K. forces his attentions on Dora, Freud clearly sympathizes with him, regarding her behavior rather than his as inappropriate. When Herr K. maneuvers Dora into a situation in which he can embrace her without fear of observation, Freud comments: "This was surely just the situation to call up a distinct feeling of sexual excitement in a girl of fourteen who had never before been approached."[9] Freud interprets her failure to experience excitement as evidence of her hysteria.

In this scene—second in order of mention, but first in order of time—the behavior of this child of fourteen was already entirely and completely hysterical. I should without question consider a person hysterical in whom an occasion for sexual excitement elicited feelings that were preponderantly or exclusively unpleasurable; and I should do so whether or no the person were capable of producing somatic symptoms. (*SE* 7:28; *C* 44)

Later, referring to the scene by the lake in which Herr K. propositions Dora, Freud observes: "Her behavior must have seemed as incomprehensible to the man after she had left him as to us, for he must long before have gathered from innumerable small signs that he was secure of the girl's affections" (*SE* 7:46; *C* 63).

Freud sees both incidents through the eyes of Herr K., going as far as to provide Herr K. with an erection at the scene of the kiss.[10] The origin of this fantasy, however justified, is clearly signaled in the following passage: "I have formed in my own mind the following reconstruction of the scene. I believe that during the man's passionate embrace she felt not merely his kiss upon her lips but also the pressure of his erect member against her body" (*SE* 7:30; *C* 47). On the basis of this fantasy, Freud concludes that Dora's feelings of disgust represents a displacement upward of a sensation on the lower part of her body. While we have no information about the reasons for Frau K.'s preference for Dora's father as a lover, it is interesting that Freud chooses a virile construction of Herr K.'s advances. Herr K. represents in this story "normal," that is to say, aggressive male heterosexuality. By representing Dora's refusal of Herr K.'s courtship as abnormal or "hysterical," Freud protects the oedipal as opposed to the preoedipal fiction. By attempting to coerce Dora verbally into an acceptance of this structure, he further identifies with Herr K., masking his identification with Dora's father. Dora's perception that she is being handed from one man to another would seem to be accurate. The extent to which Freud occupies the role of father/seducer in this analysis appears at the end of a chain of associations linking the idea of smoke with the longing for a kiss, and Dora's thumb sucking to the desire on her part for a kiss from him. "I came to the conclusion that the idea had probably occurred to her one day during a session that she would like to have a kiss from me" (*SE* 7:74; *C* 92).

If we examine Freud's line of argument as the product of *his* unconscious needs and wishes, applying his own interpretive rules to his narrative, we arrive at a view of this case history as an attempted seduction via interpretation. From this point of view, moreover, many of Freud's digressions and overstatements make sense as expressions not of his scientific neutrality but of his anxiety.

The Rights of the Gynecologist. It is axiomatic for Freud, in his analysis of Dora's motives, that "there is no such thing at all as an unconscious "No" (*SE* 7:57; *C* 75). Denial, from this vantage point, may be interpreted as affirmation: "If this 'No,' instead of being regarded as the expression of an impartial judgement (of which, indeed, the patient is incapable), is ignored, and if work is continued, the first evidence soon begins to appear that in such a case 'No' signifies the desired 'Yes' " (*SE* 7:58-59; *C* 76). Freud's rule for interpreting accusations, moreover, is to look for self-reproaches: "A string of reproaches against other people leads one to suspect the existence of a string of self-reproaches with the same content. All that need be done is to turn back each particular reproach onto the speaker himself" (*SE* 7:35; *C* 51).

With these two principles in mind, one may interpret Freud's furious denial of the charge of titillating his patient with sexual language, coupled with his anxiety about being reproached, as an indication that he is doing just that.[11] Freud's attempts to disarm such criticism, tend only, moreover, to make matters worse. In anticipating the astonishment and horror of his readers at his attribution of the fantasy of fellatio to Dora, he first appeals to the analogy of the gynecologist. Claiming that it is possible for a man to speak to young women about sexual matters "without doing them harm and without bringing suspicion on himself," he argues, "A gynaecologist, after all, under the same conditions, does not hesitate to make them submit to uncovering every possible part of their body" (*SE* 7:48; *C* 65), thus introducing new associations concerning nudity.[12] Next, in defense of the use of technical language to describe sexual matters, he falls into a syntactical slip whereby he seems to be saying that if a woman is ignorant of certain physiological processes, he instructs her concerning them: "I call bodily organs and processess by their technical names, and I tell these to the patient if they—the names, I mean—happen to be unknown to her" (*SE* 7:48; *C* 65).

As if to compound this error, he concludes, appealing to the euphemistic idiom of another language, "J'appelle un chat un chat."[13] Continuing in this vein, and introducing another set of unwanted associations, he argues that "pour faire une omelette il faut casser des oeufs." If something is to be broken, it would seem to be Dora's innocence. "There is never any danger of corrupting an innocent girl," Freud affirms. "For where there is no knowledge of sexual processes even in the unconscious, no hysterical symptom will arise; and where hysteria is found there can no longer be any question of 'innocence of mind' in the sense in which parents and educators use the phrase" (*SE* 7:49; *C* 66).

Having metaphorically undressed and violated Dora, Freud then declares her to be experienced already, a kind of Victorian Lolita, whose early pleasure in thumb sucking is cited as evidence of her predisposition toward the fantasy of "sucking at the male organ" (*SE* 7:51; *C* 68).[14] Freud's own ambivalence about this fantasy, reflected in part in his indulgence in this digression, appears as well in his classification of fellatio as one of the "aberrations of the sexual instincts" and in his need to defend himself for not taking "every opportunity of inserting into the text expressions of his personal repugnance at such revolting things" (*SE* 7:50; *C* 67). The question may well be not what Dora wanted from Freud but what he wanted from her.

While Freud attributes Dora's unwillingness to continue therapy with him to a desire for revenge, arguing on the basis of her identification with the rejected governess, he does not perceive the extent to which he stands in the position of the spurned lover, or the extent to which he may share her feelings of betrayal and consequent desire for retaliation.[15] At the same time, he feels the need to defend himself from the reproach of betraying her by writing her history.

> I shall not escape blame by this means. Only, whereas before I was accused of giving no information about my patients, now I shall be accused of giving information about my patients which ought not be given. I can only hope that in both cases the critics will be the same, and that they will merely have shifted the pretext for their reproaches. (*SE* 7:7; *C* 21)

Reading this statement, once again, in the context of Freud's interpretations of Dora's reproaches and denials, one arrives at a self-reproach on Freud's part for wishing to expose and humiliate his client. Such a desire—to pain Dora—appears at the end of a statement assuring the reader of her anonymity.

> I naturally cannot prevent the patient herself from being pained if her own case history should accidentally fall into her hands. But she will learn nothing from it that she does not already know: and she may ask herself who besides her could discover from it that she is the subject of this paper. (*SE* 7:8-9; *C* 23)

The callousness of this remark immediately supplemented by Freud's other invocation of the rights of the gynecologist suggests that he fully intends to bare Dora's secrets and to reveal her intimacies in a manner that would hurt her. Anticipating a reproach concerning his frank discussion of sexual matters, he says:

> Am I, then, to defend myself upon this score as well? I will simply claim for myself the rights of the gynaecologist—or rather, much more modest ones—and add that it would be the mark of a singular and perverse prurience to suppose that conversations of this kind are a good means of exciting or of gratifying sexual desires. (*SE* 7:9; *C* 23)

In view of Freud's understanding of writing as a supplement for Herr K.'s absence, it does not seem unreasonable to consider the supplementary functions of either conversation or the writing of a case history.[16]

The interpretation of Dora's two dreams serves at least two functions, that of oedipal camouflage for a preoedipal fantasy based on the figure of the nurse and that of revenge. It is the combination of these two elements that accounts, I believe, for the coercive quality of Freud's interpretations and for the uneasy tone of the narrative. In his relentless pursuit of a heterosexual interpretation of Dora's desire, Freud often substitutes his own train of associations for hers, a tactic that reveals the extent to which he idealizes the figure of Herr K. in order to blame Dora for her refusal. On an interpretive level, he subjects her to a process of defloration, impregnation, and parturition in an aggressively oedipal fashion, at the same time that he invalidates her rejection by naming it hysteria. Metaphorically, Freud seems to accomplish what he cannot in fact, neatly turning the tables on Dora by seducing and abandoning her, revealing in the process her "dirty secrets," her habit of masturbation and her catarrh. Thus discredited and shamed, the nurse/nursemaid/governess is deprived of her power.

The logic Freud pursues in his interpretation of Dora's first dream leads him to accuse her of childhood masturbation (hardly a remarkable discovery), the repudiation of which then provides him with evidence of her repressed desire for Herr K.

For if Dora felt unable to yield to her love for the man, if in the end she repressed that love instead of surrendering to it, there was no factor upon which her decision depended more directly than upon her premature sexual enjoyment and its consequences—her bed-wetting, her catarrh, and her disgust. (*SE* 7:87; *C* 107)

As if to underscore this point, Freud repeats:

There was a conflict within her between a temptation to yield to the man's proposal and a composite force rebelling against that feeling. This latter force was made up of motives of respectability and good sense, of hostile feelings caused by the governess's disclosures (jealousy and wounded pride, as we shall see later), and of a neurotic element, namely, the tendency to a repudiation of sexuality which was already present in her and was based on her childhood history. (*SE* 7:88; *C* 108)

The reasoning by which Freud arrives at this conclusion, however, is highly questionable, based as it is on his own verbal conversions and the presumption of causal relationships between masturbation, bed-wetting, and vaginal discharge.

It is the element of fire, of course, in Dora's first dream, that leads to the speculations about bed-wetting, through Freud's own associations to the phrase "something might happen in the night so that it might be necessary to leave the room" (*SE* 7:65; *C* 82), and his folkloristic explanation of the parental prohibition against playing with matches, an explanation of which Dora, by the way, seems to be ignorant.

She knew nothing about it.—Very well, then; the fear is that if they do they will wet their bed. The antithesis of "water" and "fire" must be at the bottom of this. Perhaps it is believed that they will dream of fire and then try and put it out with water. I cannot say exactly. (*SE* 7:72; *C* 89)

Having established his own conviction that where there is fire there must be water, Freud presumes a history of bed-wetting in Dora's family. While adapted to his dream theory, which he wishes to elucidate by means of Dora, this piece of information would seem to be irrelevant to her present condition, were it not for the spurious connection between bed-wetting and masturbation, subsequently affirmed by Freud: "Bed-wetting of this kind has, to the best of my knowledge, no more likely cause than masturbation, a habit whose importance in the aetiology of bed-wetting in general is still insufficiently appreciated" (*SE* 7:74; *C* 92).

Masturbation itself would seem equally irrelevant were it not for Freud's medically unsupported notion of a causal relation between masturbation and vaginal discharge.

> I met her half-way by assuring her that in my view the occurrence of leucorrhoea in young girls pointed primarily to masturbation, and I considered that all the other causes which were commonly assigned to that complaint were put in the background by masturbation. I added that she was now on the way to finding an answer to her own question of why it was that precisely she had fallen ill—by confessing that she had masturbated, probably in childhood. (*SE* 7:76; *C* 94)

Dora's discharge is then cited as further evidence of the preferred fantasy of fellatio: "It came to represent sexual intercourse with her father by means of Dora's identifying herself with Frau K." (*SE* 7:83; *C* 102). If Freud seeks to win an admission from Dora that she masturbated in childhood, moreover, it is because such an admission constitutes a preliminary surrender to the heterosexual solution proposed for hysteria.[17]

> Hysterical symptoms hardly ever appear so long as children are masturbating, but only afterwards, when a period of abstinence has set in; they form a substitute for masturbatory satisfaction, the desire for which continues to persist in the unconscious until another and more normal kind of satisfaction appears—where that is still attainable. For upon whether it is still attainable or not depends the possibility of a hysteria being cured by marriage and normal sexual intercourse. (*SE* 7:79; *C* 97–8)

With this interpretive frame, Freud construes Dora's melancholy dream of rescue (in which the very man to whom she appeals for protection is in the act of betraying her) as a statement of repressed desire. If she perceives her jewel-case to be in danger, not only of being wetted but of being contaminated by the veneral diseases that seem to circulate in this domestic daisy chain, it is neither her father nor her analyst who is likely to help her, since both are driving her into the arms of Herr K. It is hardly surprising that her second dream seems dominated by a mood of confusion and that the figure eliminated in this dream is that of the father.

As Dora stiffens against Freud's attempts to persuade her of her desire to be violated by Herr K., Freud becomes more entrenched in his insistence that she fantasizes not only fellatio and intercourse but also impregnation, following once again his own train of association. It is for Freud that the words *Bahnhof*, a place of commerce, and *Friedhof*, a place of death, are suggestive of female genitals, and it is he who supplies the additional term *Vorhof* as the link with nymphae, a term uncommon even among physicians for the labia minora. Instead of questioning the capacity of an eighteen-year-old girl to reproduce this series, he argues backward that she must have derived such arcane knowledge from books, "and not from popular ones either, but from anatomical text-books or from an encyclopedia—the common refuge of youth when it is devoured by sexual curiosity" (*SE* 7:99; *C* 120). He concludes, ignoring the implications of his own intrusiveness, that her dream represents a "phantasy of defloration, the phantasy of a man seeking to force an entrance into the female genitals" (*SE* 7:100; *C* 120). A truly ingenious argument follows in which Freud manages to convert a presumed attack of appendicitis accompanied by a fever and an injury to Dora's foot into hysterical symptoms representing a "phantasy of childbirth." Triumphantly, then, he concludes:

> If it is true that you were delivered of a child nine months after the scene by the lake, and that you are going about to this very day carrying the consequences of your false step with you, then it follows that in your unconscious you must have regretted the upshot of the scene. (*SE* 7:103-104; *C* 124–25)

All paths lead to Herr K., whom Freud fantastically imagines as an appropriate suitor with honorable intentions (*SE* 7:108; *C* 130). Trapped in this interpretive labyrinth, "Dora disputed the fact no longer" (*SE* 7:104; *C* 125).

Given Freud's bias in favor of Herr K. as an unconventional though perfectly acceptable lover, he can only interpret Dora's resistance as "a morbid craving for revenge" and her rejection of her treatment as an "unmistakable act of vengeance." Revealing his own wounded feelings, however, he describes the effect of Dora's "breaking off so unexpectedly, just when my hopes of a successful termination of the treatment were at their highest," as "bringing those hopes to nothing" (*SE* 7:109; *C* 131). If Dora, in the one gesture permitted the figure with whom she had been identified (the governess), wishes to injure Freud, she seems to be successful: "For how could the patient take a more effective revenge than by demonstrating upon her own person the helplessness and incapacity of the physician" (*SE* 7:120; *C* 142).

Dora's flight leaves Freud to wrestle with the specters of self-doubt and impotence, an implicit identification not with the supposedly virile Herr K. but with the invalid father. Freud's attempted camouflage of this figure through his aggressively heterosexual interpretation of Dora's desire is unmasked by her noncooperation. In the face of this refusal, he can only insist repeatedly that she is in error. His own self-justification, as well as his revenge, takes the form of a lonely monologue in which he exposes and shames the lost object of his desire—her absence providing both the animus for his narrative and its ultimate irresolution.[18]

HYSTERICAL NARRATIVE

Among the symptoms of hysteria, Freud points to the patients' inability to produce a "smooth and precise" history.

> They can, indeed, give the physician plenty of coherent information about this or that period of their lives; but it is sure to be followed by another period as to which their communications run dry, leaving gaps unfilled, and riddles unanswered; and then again will come yet another period which will

remain totally obscure and unilluminated by even a single piece of serviceable information. (*SE* 7:16; *C* 30)

From this point of view, it is the goal of analysis to restore or to construct "an intelligible, consistent, and unbroken case history" (*SE* 7:18; *C* 32). Given this understanding, Freud's "Fragment of an Analysis of a Case of Hysteria" appears to be structured around a central irony—the attempt to complete a story and to achieve narrative closure rendered forever impossible through Dora's deliberate rupture. Freud's claim that the case would have been fully elucidated had Dora stayed only underscores its actual state of incompletion.

The treatment was not carried through to its appointed end, but was broken off at the patient's own wish when it had reached a certain point. At that time some of the problems of the case had not even been attacked and others had only been imperfectly elucidated; whereas if the work had been continued we should no doubt have obtained the fullest possible enlightenment upon every particular of the case. In the following pages, therefore, I can present only a fragment of an analysis. (*SE* 7:12; *C* 26)

Not only does Freud begin his case history with a statement about its "ungratifying conclusion," he also finds occasion periodically to remind the reader of its deficiencies: "I should like to be able to add some definite information as to when and under what particular influence Dora gave up masturbating; but owing to the incompleteness of the analysis I have only fragmentary material to present" (*SE* 7:79; *C* 98).

The gaps in Freud's own narrative cause him to resort to "guessing and filling in what the analysis offers him in the shape of hints and allusions" (*SE* 7:42; *C* 58). Yet, he assures the reader: "It is only because the analysis was prematurely broken off that we have been obliged in Dora's case to resort to framing conjectures and filling in deficiencies. Whatever I have brought forward for filling up the gaps is based upon other cases which have been more thoroughly analysed" (*SE* 7:85, *C* 104).

Freud's anxiety about filling gaps coupled with his awareness of the impossibility of constructing a seamless case history reveal the extent to which he participates in the phenomenon he describes as hysterical narrative. As if to emphasize his failure to achieve closure, he writes the last section as a "postscript," beginning it with yet another statement of inadequacy: "It is true that I have introduced this paper as a fragment of an analysis; but the reader will have discovered that it is incomplete to a far greater degree than its title might have led him to expect" (*SE* 7:112; *C* 133).

In a structural sense, Freud's insistence on the fragmentary nature of his narrative, and in particular on his inability to fill all the gaps, points to the failure of his interpretation, to the failure of his verbal seduction of Dora, whom he imagines at one point as a wholly intractable subject and whose behavior he views as a rejection of all men. "Men are all so detestable that I would rather not marry. This is my revenge" (*SE* 7:120; *C* 142). Freud, in his pursuit of a phallic interpretation of Dora's desire, urging her toward a heterosexual pact in which her gap will be filled and his case history brought to a suitable conclusion, does not perceive the way in which phallic aggressiveness itself acts as a symptom. If writing may be viewed as a supplement, then the fragmentation of Freud's narrative attests not only to the impossibility of this task but also to the anxiety it generates in him. Freud's interpretive choices—fellatio over cunnilingus, the virility of Herr K. in contrast to the impotence of Dora's father, and an identification with the master rather than the governess—all point to the source of this anxiety as female identification.

What many critics, both feminist and nonfeminist, have found conspicuously wanting in this case history is any consistent portrayal of Dora's dilemma from her point of view. Standing in the way of Freud's ability to identify with Dora, I believe, are two sets of associations: one that equates femininity with castration, so that a man occupying a passive, submissive, or feminine position in a sexual relation is subject to the anxiety of castration; and another that equates female sexuality in its clitoral manifestations with the rejection of heterosexual intercourse.[19] These two sets of associations appear symptomatically in the narrative in the references to bisexuality and homosexuality, which Freud mentions as asides, never integrating them into his main arguments concerning Dora.[20] The reference to bisexuality, the most threatening to Freud's concept of aggressive male heterosexuality, occurs at the end of a list of topics which he declines to develop: "But once again in the present paper I have not gone fully into all that might be said to-day about 'somatic compliance,' about the infantile germs of perversion, about the erotogenic zones, and about our predisposition towards bisexuality" (*SE* 7:113-114; *C* 135).

When Freud refers to the possibly homosexual element in Dora's relationship with Frau K., he does so as an afterthought at the end of a chapter, making a significant association, moreover, between female homosexuality and masculinity: "These masculine or, more properly speaking, gynaecophilic currents of feeling are to be regarded as typical of the unconscious life of hysterical girls" (*SE* 7:63; *C* 81). The most notable reference to female homosexuality appears oddly in a footnote: "I failed to discover in time and to inform the patient that her homosexual (gynaecophilic) love for Frau K. was the strongest unconscious current in her mental life" *(SE 7:120n.; C 142n.)*.

The allusions to both bisexuality and homosexuality, on the margins of the narrative, as it were, and hence only partially repressed, raise again the question of what is accomplished by Freud's rather shrill insistence on Dora's love for Herr K. The fantasy of vaginal penetration functions in this case history, I think, in two ways: it both allays and maintains the anxiety of castration, as it both permits and denies a fantasy of male passivity. It functions on the one hand as a sign of virility and a means of filling a gap, of confronting and defeating the fear provoked by the sight of a woman's genitals, at the same time that it establishes a dominant–submissive relation in which a woman's "masculine" autoerotic power is denied. While Freud wishes to maintain the sexually indeterminate position of a Herr K. in the fantasy of fellatio, he simultaneously wants to divorce it from associations with male homosexuality and to eliminate the power of the nurse. In order to do this, however, he must win Dora's assent. By withholding that gratification, Dora not only holds out for the possibility of another interpretation of femininity but also stands as a silent witness to the anxieties and repressions of Freud's narrative.

Freud's attempt to enforce an oedipal interpretation on Dora's desire coupled with his repeated attempts to achieve narrative closure point finally to a fear associated with that of castration, although not identified with it: that of not being in control. Above all, perhaps, he wishes not to *be* Dora, the victim of multiple betrayals and subject to everyone's desire but her own. Against her silence, his simulated conversations sound awkward, a manic insistence on the power of *his* voice to create her reality. Finally, however, he does not even have the power of a Pygmalion to make a woman who will love him. She is more like Spenser's False Florimell, a seductive but empty image, composed literally of dead metaphors. Surely at least the misunderstandings of female sexuality prevalent at the turn of the century, the misnamings of the sources of female pleasure, are by now dead metaphors. Freud's own anxieties and confusions regarding the nonreproductively oriented nature of female sexuality, although not unusual for his time, provide, however, an insuperable barrier to a noncoercive representation not only of heterosexual intercourse but also of any kind of adult sexual encounter. What he repeatedly misses is the other clue tantalizingly offered in his choice of a name for Dora, a clue that haunts and eludes him throughout his distraught narrative—the vision of sexual relations as open to vulnerability and to risk.[21] If the indeterminacy of sex roles, like the indeterminacy of narrative form, represents a state of not being in control, then it is no surprise that Freud is unable to imagine love as something not taken but given.

Still at the heart of his naming of Dora lies another possibility, that of a love unbound by the conventions of comic narrative (which traditionally closes with marriage), the possibility of a love mutually desired and mutually gratifying, revealed in the Greek root of her name—like an open secret perhaps, but an as yet unopened gift.

Notes

1. There is an extremely rich body of commentary on *Dora*. Many readers who have found themselves entangled in this case history have pointed to areas of Freud's own unacknowledged entanglement in Dora's dilemma. The following sources find varying degrees of sexual interest on the part of Freud toward his young and attractive patient and corresponding feelings of anger and pain at her noncooperation with the treatment and her subsequent departure: essays 3, 6, 8, and 11 in this book; Lewin, Malcolm, Muslin and Gill, and Rogow in the Bibliography. While these read-

ers stress Freud's implicit alliance with Herr K. in his libidinal involvement with Dora, other commentators suggest an identification with Dora herself—with her hysteria. See essays 5, 7, and 10 in this book.

2. Steven Marcus, *Representations: Essays on Literature and Society* (New York: Random House, 1976), p. 309. Exploring the implications of the choice of the name Dora, Marcus reminds us: "Dora, of course, was David Copperfield's first love and first wife. She is at once a duplication of David's dead mother and an incompetent and helpless creature, who asks David to call her his 'child-wife.' She is also doomed not to survive, and Dickens kills her off so David can proceed to realize himself in a fuller way. One could go on indefinitely with such analogies, but the point should be sufficiently clear: in the very name he chose, Freud was true to his method, theory, and mind, expressing the overdeterminations and ambivalences that are so richly characteristic of this work as a whole."

I have taken Marcus' essay, in which he regards the writing of a case history as an instance of modern narrative, and Freud himself as a typical "unreliable narrator," as a model for my own mode of investigation, treating both Freud and Dora as characters in a novella authored by Freud himself. While I recognize the necessary distance between any author and his self-representations, I am taking the liberty psychoanalytic critics usually allow themselves of exploring the psychological implications of certain narrative and rhetorical forms. More precisely, I have taken Freud's own theoretical pronouncements about Dora and used them to illustrate his portrait of himself.

3. Arnold Rogow provides some interesting historical information about the Bauer household, including some details of Käthe Bauer's concern for cleanliness. The most extensive treatment of the background of the Bauer family that I have encountered, however, is provided by Maria Ramas in the unabridged version of the essay in this book. Iza Erlich discusses the difference between Freud's vivid treatment of the men in this case history and that of Dora's mother, whom he dismisses rather summarily. She concludes: "It is as if Freud could not bring himself to look closely at the mother, the figure his theory proclaims to be so central. Be it Dora's madly cleaning mother, Little Hans' beautiful, seductive mother, or the Rat Man's absentee mother, they all appear as silhouettes against the rich background of other relationships, other entanglements." See "What Happened to Jocasta," *Bulletin of the Menninger Clinic* (1977), 41:284.

The way in which Freud subordinates Dora's mother may be related to his sketchy treatment of the homosexual element in Dora's affectional life, an element that embraces not only her avowed love for Frau K. but also her apparently conflicted feelings toward her mother. Among critics who touch on this subject are Karl Kay Lewin, Toril Moi, Philip Rieff, and Maria Ramas.

4. The figure of the nursemaid, whose position as servant, surrogate mother, and sexual object in the Victorian household makes her the locus of exploitation, regressive fantasy, and desire, is central to this case history. Critics who have commented

on the family structures and erotic implications of the inclusion of such a figure in the Victorian family are the following: Leonore Davidoff, "Class and Gender in Victorian England: The Diaries of Arthur J. Munby and Hannah Cullwick," *Feminist Studies* (1979), 5:87–141; Sander Gilman, "Freud and the Prostitute: Male Stereotypes of Female Sexuality in fin de siècle Vienna," *Journal of the American Academy of Psychoanalysis* (1981), 9(3):337–60; Theresa McBride, "As the Twig Is Bent: The Victorian Nanny," in Anthony S. Wohl ed., *The Victorian Family: Structure and Stresses*, pp. 44–58 (New York: St. Martin's Press, 1978); and Maria Ramas. Jim Swan, in a remarkable essay entitled "Mater and Nannie: Freud's Two Mothers and the Discovery of the Oedipus Complex," *American Imago* (1974), 31:1–64, explores the origin in Freud's own infancy of the image of the woman split into the idealized mother and the debased object of desire. Kenneth Griggs points out the ways in which the figure of Freud's nursemaid and his mother are conflated in some of his dreams in "All Roads Lead to Rome: The Role of the Nursemaid in Freud's Dreams," *Journal of the American Psychoanalytic Association* (1973), 21:108–26. Jane Gallop argues that class difference (as well as sexual difference) prevents Freud from being able to identify with the figure of the governess. See essay 10 in this book.

5. The line of reasoning here is that Dora's use of the word *vermögender*, which has connotations of sexual potency, reveals the true nature of Dora's thought, which is just the opposite. It does not seem to occur to Freud to wonder how Dora might have come by such knowledge of her father's prowess or lack of it. Here as elsewhere Freud's verbal preoccupations are evident.

6. While the subject of Dora's and Frau K.'s reading may never be fully elucidated, it seems clear to me from my reading of Paolo Mantegazza's *The Physiology of Love* that Dora would not have obtained knowledge of specific sexual practices therefrom. *The Physiology of Love* (published in 1877), one of a trilogy of books by Mantegazza dealing with human sexuality, is largely a romantic and sentimental paen to human reproduction. See *The Physiology of Love*, Herbert Alexander, tr., Victor Robinsin, ed. (New York: Eugenics, 1936). If on the other hand Dora had read the more explicit text by Mantegazza, *The Sexual Relations of Mankind*, then she would have discovered a full sexual vocabulary including references to lesbian lovemaking. Critics who have noted the oddness of Freud's choice of fellatio over cunnilingus are Neil Hertz and Toril Moi, as well as Sharon Willis, "A Symptomatic Narrative," *Diacritics* (Spring 1983), pp. 46–60. Willis relates Freud's "blindness" in this instance to the phallocentrism of his discourse.

7. Others have proposed different reasons for Freud's avoidance of the feminine position. See in particular the essays by Jane Gallop, Neil Hertz, and Jerre Collins et al. in this book.

8. See *SE* 7:28–9; *C* 43–44. It is perhaps not surprising that Freud was predisposed in favor of Herr K., given the fact that it was he who introduced Dora's father to Freud for the treatment of syphilis.

9. Several critics have commented on the inappropriateness of Freud's expectation

that Dora should have been aroused. Erik Erikson, Mark Kanzer, Steven Marcus, Toril Moi, and Philip Rieff all signal Freud's failure to take into account the full complexity of Dora's dilemma, including the fact of her adolescence. See Erikson's essay in this book and Kanzer's "The Motor Sphere of the Transference," in Bibliography.

I find Marcus' statement in essay 3 of this volume describing Dora's situation in many ways the most poignant and acute: "The three adults to whom she was closest, whom she loved the most in the world, were apparently conspiring—separately, in tandem, or in concert—to deny Dora her reality and reality itself. This betrayal touched upon matters that might easily unhinge the mind of a young person; the three adults were not betraying Dora's love and trust alone, they were betraying the structure of the actual world."

Maria Ramas calls the process by which Dora's version of events was either undermined or denied "gaslighting." If subsequent accounts of Dora's life are true (see, for example, Felix Deutsch, essay 1 of this book), the "success" of Freud's treatment may be gauged by Dora's inability either to throw off her neurosis or to accept the terms within which Freud offered cure.

10. Toril Moi states, "It is little wonder that he [Freud] feels the need to defend himself against the idea of fellatio, since it is more than probable that the fantasy exists, not in Dora's mind, but in his alone" (see essay 8).

11. Jerre Collins et al. also make this point in essay 11 of this book.

12. Mary Daly has also noticed the intrusive and prurient implications of this statement. See *Gyn/Ecology* (Boston: Beacon Press, 1978), p. 256.

13. See Jane Gallop's essay in this volume for a particularly witty discussion of this resort to euphemism.

14. Sander Gilman finds ample evidence in nineteenth-century Vienna of the stereotype of female children as sexually precocious. He links this attitude to the prevalence of adolescent prostitutes, the exploitation of lower-class women generally, and the need of their male clients to "blame the victim." He speculates that Freud's ideas concerning the seductiveness of children may derive in part from prevailing stereotypes of female sexuality and in part from his own need to deny parental seduction of female children. From this point of view one may well ask to what extent Freud projects his own sexual desires onto Dora.

15. For Toril Moi, Freud's revenge consists in part of his fixing Ida Bauer with the name of his sister's servant. See essay 8 this volume.

16. I am using "supplement" in the Derridean sense as both an attempt to fill a void, to create a presence, and as an inevitable reminder of a void or an absence. I am guided here by Freud's own observation that Dora took up her pen when Herr K. was absent. Toril Moi, discussing the "supplementary" status of Freud's text, states, "Freud's text oscillates endlessly between his desire for complete insight or knowledge and an unconscious realization (or fear) of the fragmentary, deferring status of knowledge itself."

17. Freud's views on the relationship between masturbation and hysteria are not unusual for his time, nor is his assumption that heterosexual intercourse offers a cure. Richard Krafft-Ebing, whom Freud most assuredly read, is unequivocal in his conviction that masturbation poses an obstacle to heterosexual relations. See *Psychopathia Sexualis,* Harry E. Wedeck, tr. (New York: Putnam, 1965). While less virulent on this subject, Freud is entirely conventional in his assumption that masturbation for women must be abandoned and replaced by heterosexual intercourse to ensure normal female development. Paolo Mantegazza, perhaps not incidentally, in *The Sexual Relations of Mankind,* adopts the same view. For feminist critiques of the compulsory and institutionalized nature of heterosexuality in patriarchal culture, see Maria Ramas' essay in this volume, and Adrienne Rich, "Compulsory Heterosexuality and Lesbian Existence," *Signs* (1980), 5:631–659. For speculations about the social environment that defined nineteenth-century conceptions of hysteria, see Roberta Satow, "Where Has All the Hysteria Gone," *Psychoanalytic Review* (1979–80), 66:463–473; and Carol Smith-Rosenberg, "The Hysterical Woman: Sex Roles and Role Conflict in 19th Century America," *Social Research* (1972), 39:652–78.

18. I am indebted to Sara Eaton for this insight. In "A Symptomatic Narrative," Sharon Willis describes Dora's disruptive status as a refusal "to enter the system of circulation governed by the phallus as master signifier." See *Diacritics* (Spring 1983), p. 47.

19. Freud's insistence that the clitoris is a masculine organ and that the little girl's pleasure in it is phallic creates an insuperable barrier to his understanding of female sexuality as anything but an obstacle to the achievement of heterosexual intercourse. He must at some level have understood that he was fighting a losing battle in trying to convince his female patients to abandon this obvious source of pleasure. Paolo Mantegazza, who seems on the whole less conflicted about this subject, nevertheless is clear in his assumption that a woman who has become accustomed to clitoral stimulation will require her lover to learn how to satisfy her in this way.

20. For alternate explanations of Freud's nervous treatment of bisexuality and homosexuality, see the essays by Jerre Collins et al., and by Jane Gallop in this volume, and Willis, "A Symptomatic Narrative."

21. Janet Malcolm's suggestion that "Dora" refers ultimately to the Pandora of mythology is altogether convincing I think. I would only like to add that in its simplest form "Dora" refers to the "gift" that Freud could neither acknowledge nor accept. For him the encounter with this attractive and intelligent woman was always a power struggle of sorts, never an exchange of vulnerabilities. In this sense "Dora" stands for all that Freud could neither understand nor simply allow to *be* on its own terms in the other sex.

Bibliography

The following bibliography is limited to works devoted either entirely or in significant part to the Dora case. Studies reprinted in this book are not listed. For a bibliography that includes books and articles concerned in a more general way with the issues the case raises (and to which we are greatly indebted), see the issue of *Diacritics* cited below.

COLLECTIONS

Revue française de psychanalyse (1973), vol. 37, no. 3. This issue is devoted to Dora. It includes the following articles, introduced by the editor, René Major:

René Major. "L'hystérie: Rêve et révolution." A translation of this article, entitled "The Revolution in Hysteria," is available in the *International Journal of Psychoanalysis* 55 (1974), 385–392, where it is accompanied by a "Discussion" by C. David.

Ilana Schimmel, "Rêve et transfert dans 'Dora.' "

Claude Hollande. "A propos de l'identification hystérique."

Evelyne Ville. "Analité et hystérie."

Dominique J. Geahchan. "Haine et identification négative dans l'hystérie."

Jean-Jacques Moscovitz. "D'un signe qui lui serait fait, ou aspects de l'homosexualité dans 'Dora.' " Abstract in *Psychoanalytic Quarterly* 45 (1976).

Jacqueline Lubtchansky. "Le point de vue économique dans l'hystérie à partir de la notion de traumatisme dans l'oeuvre de Freud."

Mark Kanzer and Jules Glenn, eds., *Freud and His Patients.* New York: Aronson, 1980.

Includes a section of interpretations by analysts of the Dora case:

Jules Glenn. "Notes on Psychoanalytic Concepts and Style in Freud's Case Histories."

—— "Freud's Adolescent Patients: Katharina, Dora and the 'Homosexual Woman.' "

Melvin A. Scharfman. "Further Reflections on Dora."
Robert J. Langs. "The Misalliance Dimension in the Case of Dora."
Mark Kanzer. "Dora's Imagery: The Flight from a Burning House."
Isidor Bernstein. "Integrative Summary: On the Re-viewings of the Dora Case."

Diacritics (Spring 1983): "A Fine Romance: Freud and Dora." Special Editor: Neil Hertz. This issue contains a translation by Sarah Burd of Hélène Cixous' play, *Portrait de Dora* (published in France by Editions des Femmes, 1976), the articles by Collins et al. and Neil Hertz reprinted here, and an article by Sharon Willis, "A Symptomatic Narrative."

OTHER WORKS

Anzieu, Didier. *L'auto-analyse de Freud et la découverte de la psychanalyse.* 2 vols. Paris: Presses Universitaires de France, 1959; rev. 1975.

Auerbach, Nina. *Woman and the Demon: The Life of a Victorian Myth.* Cambridge: Harvard University Press, 1982.

Benmussa, Simone. "Introduction." In *Benmussa Directs.* London: Calder, 1979.

Blos, P. "The Epigenesis of an Adult Neurosis." *The Psychoanalytic Study of the Child* (1972), no. 27.

—— "Modifications in the Classical Psychoanalytical Model of Adolescence." *Adolescent Psychiatry* (1979), vol. 7.

Brémont, Robert. "A propos de Hans et de Dora." *Interprétation* (1968), vol. 2.

Cixous, Hélène. *Le Portrait du soleil.* Paris: Denoël, 1973.

Cixous, Hélène and Catherine Clément. *La jeune née.* Paris: 10/18, 1975. Translation forthcoming at the University of Minnesota Press.

Conley, Tom. "Fragments de Dora." *Topique* (in press).

Decker, Hannah S. "Freud and Dora: Constraints on Medical Progress." *Journal of Social History* (1981), vol. 14.

—— "The Choice of a Name: 'Dora' and Freud's Relationship with Breuer." *Journal of the American Psychoanalytic Association* (1982), vol. 30.

Erlich, Iza. "What Happened to Jocasta?" *Bulletin of the Menninger Clinic* (1977), vol. 41.

Evans, Martha Noel. "*Portrait of Dora:* Freud's Case History As Reviewed by Hélène Cixous," *Substance* (1982), no. 36.

Kanzer, Mark. "The Motor Sphere of the Transference." *Psychoanalytic Quarterly* (1966), vol. 35.

Kaplan, E. Ann. "Feminist Approaches to History, Psychoanalysis, and Cinema, in Sigmund Freud's Dora." *Millennium Film Journal* (November 1980). Also in Kaplan, *Women and Film.* New York: Methuen, 1983.

Kohon, Gregorio. "Reflections on Dora: The Case of Hysteria." *International Journal of Psycho-Analysis* (in press).

Krohn, Alan and Janis Krohn. "The Nature of the Oedipus Complex in the Dora Case." *Journal of the American Psychological Association* (1982), vol 30.

Lacan, Jacques. Brief discussions by Lacan of Dora can be found in a number of volumes of *Le Séminaire* (Paris: Seuil, 1975–):

"Les fluctuations de la libido" and "Le concept de l'analyse." In vol. 1: *Les écrits techniques de Freud* (1953–1954).

"La dissolution imaginaire," "La question hystérique," and "La question hystérique II: 'Qu'est-ce qu'une femme?' " In vol. 3: *Les psychoses* (1955–56).

"Du sujet de la certitude." In vol. 11: *Les quatres concepts fondamentaux de la psychanalyse* (1964).

Laplanche, Jean. "Panel on 'Hysteria Today.' " *International Journal of Psycho-Analysis* (1974), vol 55.

Lewin, Karl K. "Dora Revisited." *Psychoanalytic Review* (1974), vol. 60.

Lindon, J. A. "A Psychoanalytic View of the Family: A Study of Family Member Interactions." *Psychoanalytic Forum 3*. New York: International Universities Press, 1962.

Lopez, D. "Rileggendo Freud: il caso Dora." *Rivista di psicoanalisi* (1967), vol. 13.

Maddi, Salvatore R. "The Victimization of Dora." *Psychology Today* (1974), vol. 8.

Malcolm, Janet. *Psychoanalysis: The Impossible Profession*. New York: Knopf, 1981.

Manhaes, Maria. "Femininity." *Rivista Brasileira de Psicanalise* (1979), vol. 13.

Mannoni, Octave. *Fictions freudiennes*. Paris: Seuil, 1978.

Marcus, Steven. "Freud and Dora: Story, History, Case History." In *Representations*. New York: Random House, 1975. Full version of the article printed herein.

Marty, P., M. Fain, M. de M'Uzan, and Ch. David. "Le cas Dora et le point de vue psychosomatique." *Revue française de psychanalyse* (1968), vol. 32.

Matlock, Jann. "The Others of Romance: Circumventing the Proprietorship of Psychoanalysis." Ms., University of California at Berkeley, 1981.

McCaffrey, Phillip. *Freud and Dora: The Artful Dream*. Rutgers University Press, forthcoming.

McCall, Anthony and Andrew Tyndell. "Sixteen Working Statements." *Millennium Film Journal*, 1(2):29–37.

McCall, Anthony, Claire Pajaczkowska, Andrew Tyndall, and Jane Weinstock. *Sigmund Freud's Dora: A Case of Mistaken Identity*. Film 1979. Script published in *Framework* (1981), nos. 15–17, pp. 75–81.

Muslin, Hyman and Merton Gill. "Transference in the Dora Case." *Journal of the American Psychoanalytic Association* (1978), vol. 26.

Nuncio, Luz. "The Hysterical Attack: Illness as Defensive/Offensive Tactic in Dora." Ms., Yale University, 1982.

Oppé, Felicity. "Exhibiting Dora." *Screen* (1981), vol. 22.

Portuges, Catherine. "Dora in the Dark: Cinematic Deconstruction of Freud's 'Subtlest Thing.' " Forthcoming.

Ramas, Maria. "Freud's Dora, Dora's Hysteria: The Negation of a Woman's Rebellion." *Feminist Studies* (1980), vol. 6. Full version of the article printed herein.

Refabert, Philippe and Barbro Sylwan. "Dora entre Freud et Fliess." *L'Inanalysé*, Documents Confrontation, Journées de Mai 1978.

Rieff, Philip. *Fellow Teachers.* New York: Harper & Row, 1974.

Rogow, Arnold A. "A Further Footnote to Freud's 'Fragment of an Analysis of a Case of Hysteria'." *Journal of the American Psychoanalytic Association* (1978), vol. 26.

—— "Dora's Brother." *International Journal of Psychoanalysis* (1979), vol. 6.

Schlesier, Renate. *Konstruktionen der Weiblichkeit bei Sigmund Freud.* Frankfurt-am-Main: Europaiische Verlagamstatt, 1981.

Schneider, Monique. *La parole et l'inceste.* Paris: Anbier Montaigne, 1980.

Seidenberg, R. and E. Papathomopoulos. "Daughters Who Tend Their Fathers." *The Psychoanalytic Study of Society* (1962), vol. 2.

Showalter, Elaine. *The Female Malady: Women, Madness, and English Culture 1830–1980.* New York: Pantheon, forthcoming.

Slipp, Samuel. "Interpersonal Factors in Hysteria: Freud's Seduction Theory and the Case of Dora." *Journal of the American Academy of Psychoanalysis* (1977), vol. 5.

Sperling, Melitta. "Conversion Hysteria and Conversion Symptoms: A Revision of Classification and Concepts." *Journal of the American Psychoanalytic Association* (1973), vol. 21.

Spiegel, Rose. "Freud and the Women in His World." *Journal of the American Academy of Psychoanalysis* (1977), vol. 5.

Wajeman, Gérard, *Le Maître et l'hystérique.* Paris: Seuil, 1982.

Weinstock, Jane. "Sigmund Freud's Dora?" *Screen* (1981), vol. 22.

Notes on Contributors

CHARLES BERNHEIMER teaches English and Comparative Literature at the State University of New York at Buffalo and is a member of the Center for the Psychological Study of the Arts. He is the author of *Flaubert and Kafka: Studies in Psychopoetic Structure* (1982) and of numerous articles on nineteenth- and twentieth-century European literature. His current project is a book tentatively entitled "Prostitution in the Novel: Sexuality and Narrative in Nineteenth-Century France."

JERRE COLLINS teaches English at Marquette University; J. RAY GREEN is a member of the Department of Modern Foreign Languages at Boston University; ELEANOR HONIG SKOLLER and MARK SACHNER teach English at the University of Wisconsin, Milwaukee; MARY LYDON was a Fellow of the Society for the Humanities at Cornell for 1982–83. At the time the article reprinted here was composed, its authors constituted a study group at the University of Wisconsin, Milwaukee.

FELIX DEUTSCH, who died in 1964, was an eminent psychoanalyst, member of the Vienna Psychoanalytic Society, and later president of the Boston Psychoanalytic Institute, as well as a distinguished medical internist. Deutsch wrote extensively about the interrelation between psychological and physiological processes and made significant contributions to the contemporary practice of psychosomatic medicine.

ERIK ERIKSON developed through the cours of his career an epigenetic theory of identity formation that has greatly influenced both clinical practice and psychohistorical studies. After presenting a theory of ego-adaptation to stages of psychosocial development in his first book, *Childhood and Society* (1950), Erikson continued to trace the evolving relation between social structures and the human life cycle in such books as *Insight and Responsibility* (1964), *Identity: Youth and Crisis* (1968), and *Life History and the Historical Moment* (1975).

JANE GALLOP is an associate professor of French and Italian and is affiliated with Women's Studies at Miami University. A leading figure for the last decade in the movement to articulate a relation between Lacanian psychoanalysis and feminism, she has published numerous articles that try to dislodge conventional conceptions of sexual difference as well as two books: *Intersections: A Reading of Sade with Bataille, Blanchot and Klossowski* (1981); and *The Daughter's Seduction: Feminism and Psychoanalysis* (1983). She is currently at work on a critical study of Lacan's *Ecrits*.

SUZANNE GEARHART, who teaches literature at the University of California, San Diego, has published various articles on critical theory and eighteenth-century French literature. Her book, *The Open Boundary of History and Fiction: A Critical Approach to the French Enlightenment*, is forthcoming.

NEIL HERTZ, long a distinguished member of the English Department at Cornell University, is now on the faculty of the Humanities Center at Johns Hopkins University. Among his various articles, "Freud and the Sandman" and "Medusa's Head" use psychoanalysis to question textual and political strategies of interpretation. He is currently at work on a book about George Eliot. A collection of his articles is forthcoming.

CLAIRE KAHANE teaches English at the State University of New York at Buffalo and is a member of the Center for the Psychological Study of the Arts, as well as director of the literature and psychology program. The author of various psychoanalytic interpretations of British and American fiction, she has edited a collection of psychoanalytic criticism published in Germany and is coeditor, with Madelon Sprengnether and Shirley Garner, of a collection of feminist psychoanalytic essays forthcoming.

JACQUES LACAN, the French psychoanalyst who died in 1981, is one of the most controversial figures in psychoanalytic circles. Lacan charged the psychoanalytic establishment with betraying Freud's insights and set up his own school of psychoanalysis, the *école freudienne,* which he disbanded shortly before his death. In a series of seminars and papers, Lacan reformulated Freud's theory by incorporating linguistics and stressing the effects of unconscious desire. His papers are written in an elusive style that reflects his insistence on the instability of language and the division of the subject.

STEVEN MARCUS teaches English and Comparative Literature, and is George Delacorte Professor of Humanities at Columbia University. An eminent literary critic as well as a fellow of the American Psychoanalytic Association, Marcus has published numerous books, among them *The Other Victorians* (1966), an uncovering of Victorian sexuality, and a collection of essays, *Representations* (1976).

TORIL MOI was born in Norway and took her Ph.D. in French and Comparative Literature at the University of Bergen. She is currently a lecturer in French at Pembroke College, Oxford. A work-in-progress, *Sexual/Textual: An Introduction to Feminist Literary Theory,* will be published soon.

MARIA RAMAS is a doctoral candidate in the Department of History at the University of California, Los Angeles; her subject is nineteenth-century European social history. "Women's Oppression and Capitalism: A Critical Review," an article coauthored with Johanna Brenner, is forthcoming in *New Left Review.* Her current project is a study of the social bases of conversion hysteria in nineteenth-century Europe.

JACQUELINE ROSE teaches literature at the University of Sussex, England, and is the coeditor, with Juliet Mitchell, of a collection of Lacanian essays, *Feminine Sexuality: Jacques Lacan and the Ecole Freudienne* (1983). She is currently completing a book, *The Case of Peter Pan or the Impossibility of Children's Fiction.*

MADELON SPRENGNETHER, formerly Madelon Gohlke, teaches English at the University of Minnesota. An active poet and essayist as well as a scholar, she has published *The Normal Heart* (1981), *Rivers, Stories, Houses, Dreams* (1983), as well as articles on Renaissance authors, and is coeditor of a forthcoming collection of feminist psychoanalytic essays tentatively entitled *The M/Other Tongue.* She is currently working on a book-length memoir, *Letter to My Daughter.*

Index

Bei Fragen zur Produktsicherheit wenden Sie sich bitte an:
If you have any questions regarding product safety,
please contact:

Walter de Gruyter GmbH
Genthiner Straße 13
10785 Berlin
productsafety@degruyterbrill.com